HEALTHY VISION

Prevent and Reverse Eye Disease through Better Nutrition

NEAL ADAMS, MD

Lyons Press
Guilford, Connecticut
Helena, Montana

An imprint of Rowman & Littlefield

Lyons Press is an imprint of Rowman & Littlefield

Distributed by NATIONAL BOOK NETWORK

British Library Cataloguing-in-Publication Information available

Library of Congress Cataloging-in-Publication Data available

ISBN 978-1-4930-0607-6 (paperback)

♾™ The paper used in this publication meets the minimum requirements of American National Standard for Information Sciences—Permanence of Paper for Printed Library Materials, ANSI/NISO Z39.48-1992.

The health information expressed in this book is not intended to be a substitute for medical advice and is not intended as a medical manual. The information should not be used for diagnosis or treatment, or as a substitute for professional medical care. You are advised not to self-diagnose and to not skip seeing your doctor. You are advised to seek medical care from a health care professional.

Dedicated to my wife and children

CONTENTS

INTRODUCTION:
OUR EYES SEE IT ALL

In good health, vision is our most important sense. Over one-third of our brain function serves our vision. So where would we be without sight? For most, our lives would be vastly different if we woke up tomorrow without our vision—a scary proposition very few will have to face. As an ophthalmologist (a physician who specializes in the anatomy, physiology, and diseases of the eye, and performs surgery on it), what I do see every day is that most of us *will* encounter—at some point in our lives—the general decline of our eyesight.

Perhaps you picked up this book because you've noticed a change in, or have developed problems with, your vision—or have a friend or family member who has. Perhaps you had to buy reading glasses for the first time, or recently realized that you can't read signs from the same distance as well as you used to. Or perhaps it's more serious—you've been recently diagnosed with cataracts, dry eye, macular degeneration, or glaucoma and aren't sure how to treat it or prevent its progress.

Regardless of why you've decided to improve your vision, this book can help you. As an ophthalmologist my passion is reading and studying the latest medical science about eye health, so I decided to make those results known and accessible to you. In this book, I'll translate the most groundbreaking clinical studies over the past few years into easy-to-implement advice that will help you maintain or perhaps even restore your vision by what you eat. Young or old—nearsighted, farsighted, or 20/20—we can all take action to help the health of our eyes.

I can gauge a patient's overall health just by looking in his or her eyes. Some say the eye is a window to the soul—as a doctor,

I know the eye is a window to the body. That's because your eyes often show how well your body is overall. The back of the eye can be the first place we as doctors see signs of many disorders such as diabetes, high blood pressure, and even life-threatening cancer, before they appear anywhere else in the body.

In fact, the earliest sign that a diabetic is developing heart disease is found by looking at blood vessels in the eye—no other blood test or scan can detect it sooner. So when I examine a patient, I can often tell who's been taking better care of his or her health. Getting the right nutrition—a healthy diet full of fruits, vegetables, fish, and whole grains—to feed your body (and your eyes) is an essential component of good health, because we truly are what we eat.

Most of what we'll talk about in this book wasn't learned in medical school, but rather from years spent practicing as an ophthalmologist and reading the latest research. Unfortunately, much of the scientific medical research—some of which is promoted in the press or to the public—is convoluted and/or misleading if not carefully understood. But embedded inside the data are clear links between eye health and nutrition, and it is this exciting avenue to health that I intend to share with you in this book.

These studies are surprisingly varied. For instance, we can learn about a link between nutrition and eye health from astronauts in outer space. In the past fifteen years, nearly forty astronauts have lived on the International Space Center for months at a time, during which time nearly 20 percent of them developed a problem with their eyes. Scientists later discovered that the astronauts who developed eye conditions had lower levels of the nutrient folate (we'll talk more about folate in chapter 4) in their bodies even though all the astronauts ate the same food (and even the same amount of that food).

It turns out the astronauts who developed eye problems had a genetically altered weak pathway in their digestive tract that caused them to absorb less folic acid and vitamin B12 (which help eye function) than their colleagues. Whereas this weak pathway may not often cause disease in regular life on the planet Earth, in outer space, it did. Though most of us aren't headed to space any time soon, it does show that changing your environment—and what you eat—can affect and even damage your eye health. And perhaps this weak pathway does affect the health of our earthbound selves in subtle ways. This book will help you identify nutritional weak links so that you can optimize the health of your eyes.

In my clinic, although I commonly get questions about whether carrots are actually good for your eyes (the answer is yes), over the years I've realized that many people don't know much more about nutrition than very basic information, let alone how specific nutrients readily found in our food can help eye health. And though I felt I was helping the patients in my office learn this information, I wanted to relay my message to every person in America concerned about their ability to see. (Which, frankly, is a lot more people than could fit in my office.)

So I wrote this book. I suspect if you've picked it up, you have already decided that you want to improve or protect your vision and eye health. Wonderful! I'm really glad for you! It's my goal to help you see your best for the rest of your life.

First, it's important to explain the inner workings of the eye before diving into the details of what damages and heals your vision. Let's learn a bit about how your eye works when all is well—before trying to fix it. After all, if you were going to fix a problem on your computer, you'd have to know how the operating system runs first—and the same applies for your body.

HOW THE EYE WORKS

The eye has many, many parts and processes, but for the purposes of this book it's only truly necessary to know the eye's major

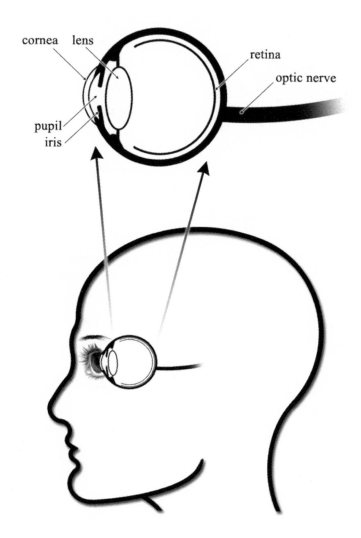

components, the ones that control your vision and are most affected by aging, environmental damage, and disease. These include the cornea, the pupil, the iris, the lens, the retina, and the optic nerve.

What you see when you look at your eyes in the mirror are the eyelids, the whites of your eyes, and (in the middle) the iris, pupil, and cornea. The pupil and iris make up what most people commonly call the eye; the pupil is the dark center and the iris is the "color" of your eye. The cornea is much less obvious; it's actually a thin layer—like a clear window—in front of the iris and pupil. If you ever see a glint or a reflection off your eye in a photograph or a mirror, you are seeing the cornea.

An easy way to understand the physical relationship between the cornea and iris is to imagine your eye as the face of a watch: the cornea is the glass, protecting the numbers and dials of the face, which is your iris and pupil. The cornea protects the inside of your eye from the outside world.

Your cornea is incredibly sensitive to touch, injury, even specks of dust. That's because there are more sensory nerve endings in the cornea per square millimeter than anywhere else in the body— which is why it hurts so darned much to get something in your eye! Though the cornea is only a half a millimeter thick, in good health it is so transparent and so perfectly curved that it can bend light and give your retina a clear view of the world around you. And, if you are healthy, your body's stem cells regenerate and replace the entire surface of your cornea every seven to ten days. It's truly an amazing part of your body.

The function of the iris and pupil is to filter the light you see by adjusting to let in more or less light. These parts of the eye function much like the aperture of a camera does. When you encounter light, the iris will dilate and constrict based on the amount of light in the environment. The pupil acts as an opening, an empty "hole" in the center of the iris, that lets light in. When you're in the dark, the pupil will enlarge to let more light in and, in sunlight, you'll notice that pupils are small, to limit the amount of light going into the eye. The iris can also dilate when you are in sudden stressful situations, as part of your flight-or-fight biological response.

Behind the iris and pupil is the lens, inside your eye. The lens focuses light to the back of your eye where the retina and optic nerve are. The lens inside your eye actually acts like a magnifying glass—ensuring that the image you see is clear and focused. This lens is the most transparent cellular tissue in the whole human body and is bathed in a fluid that is extremely rich in nutrients and vitamins.

Whereas the lens inside a camera moves back and forth to focus on an object and give you a clear picture, in the eye the lens constantly changes shape, from more curved to less curved, to give you that clear focused picture. Up to the age of about forty, the lens freely changes its shape to allow for sharp focus, depending on whether the object you are looking at is close or far away. After you reach forty, your eyes' lenses start to lose their ability to focus, and many of us have to rely on reading glasses to focus up close.

So everything we see gets focused onto the back of the eye, where the retina—a layer of light-sensing cells—creates images to send to your brain. To go back to our camera analogy, think of the retina as the photographic film of an old-model camera, or as the sensor inside a digital camera. The retina is incredibly thin, only a quarter of a millimeter, and within this quarter millimeter there are multiple layers of dozens of types of brain cells that detect light rays and process and create images that are then fed through the optic nerve to your brain. The brain interprets them, enabling you to clearly "see" around you. Controlling *where* we see are six muscles around each eyeball that help move the eyes around to whatever you want to view. These muscles are the most active muscles of your whole body!

In case you were wondering, tears aren't just for sad movies; your tears actually protect your eyes all day, every day. Tears help your eye clear out any substances (eyelashes, dust, sunscreen) that happen to work their way onto the film that covers your cornea. They are naturally antiseptic—antimicrobial—and they are full of nutrients and vitamins.

Have you ever wondered why you have to blow your nose after crying? It's because your tears don't just run down your face; there are ducts in your eye that open behind your nose and drain tears into your nose, like a gutter spout drains rainwater. That's why you should always keep a tissue at hand when watching *Schindler's List.*

HOW TO USE THIS BOOK

Obviously, this is a massively simplified version of the eye's biology and the processes that allow us to see every day. But for most people understanding how the eye works is less important than understanding what causes damage to their eyes, and how to prevent that damage over time. That's what I'll explain in the first part of this book. In the second part, I'll discuss the six main diseases that affect the eye (macular degeneration, retinitis pigmentosa, diabetes-related conditions, glaucoma, cataracts, and dry eye) from a very broad perspective. We'll talk about treatment, prevention, minimizing risk factors, and—more important—we'll discuss how understanding how each of these conditions develop allows us to improve or protect our eyesight. And, last but not least, in the third part of the book I'll synthesize all the research to provide advice on which foods can help you maintain or even improve your vision, based on whichever condition(s) you worry about. The concepts we'll learn are particularly important to me—they'll show why you simply can't make your eyes stronger by taking a pill or by solely doing eye exercises. You can, however, easily help your eyes by eating the foods that best provide the nutrients necessary for healthy vision.

A WORD ABOUT VITAMINS

Let me dispel a widely held myth: popping vitamin pills is not the same as eating foods that naturally contain vitamins and will in no way give you the same results. There are many scientific and biological reasons why this is so, but it basically comes down to potency and balance.

Since vitamins and other supplements are only loosely regulated, vitamins sold in pill form can often be more potent than necessary, which means that if you take too many too often, the vitamins will either simply pass through your body (essentially wasting your money) or accumulate to a toxic level, possibly making you very sick. Consumers are often misled into thinking more is better.

In addition, natural sources like fruits, vegetables, fish, and whole grains contain many more types of nutrients than what's found in any pill. This broad variety of nutrients will interact with each other and support each other in a more harmonious balance than a combination of pills will. And, in most places, purchasing seasonal produce is cheaper than heading to the vitamin aisle for the same nutrient in a bottle. I believe—and advise all my patients—that it's better both for your body and your wallet to get your vitamins by eating fresh food than by swallowing a pill.

THE IMPORTANCE OF NUTRITION

You will notice throughout the book that I believe the primary tool to prevent and treat vision problems is proper nutrition. But it isn't just me. After reading the results of clinical trials and other articles by doctors and researchers in medical journals, and learning from my patients throughout the years, the evidence clearly points to a link between nutrition and eye health. I will synthesize what I've learned from these sources throughout this book. You can trust that all my recommendations and information, dietary and otherwise, come from a valid scientific study or source (citations are listed in the bibliography for your use and reference in conversations with your doctor).

Before I begin, I'd like to be clear that I do not believe there is ever a one-size-fits-all solution for your health, or for your vision. As with most things in life, when it comes to your sight and this book you should implement what applies to you, use what works for you, and leave the rest behind. Most important, you need to work closely with your doctor, who knows your medical needs the best, to fine-tune your regimen and help you avoid pitfalls.

Now that we've discussed the basic functioning of the eye, the underlying research of the book, and my philosophy about how to generally approach your health, we can begin improving your vision one lesson at a time. First, you may know that getting enough oxygen is important for your lungs, but did you know that having too much oxygen in your body overall will make you feel older, faster? Read on . . .

Part I:

How to Maintain and Restore Your Vision

CHAPTER 1
THE POWER OF OXYGEN

Slice an apple and watch as the exposed flesh turns brown within minutes—you're witnessing the same process that is going on inside your body at this very moment. Also the cause of many a rusty swing set, the process is called oxidation.

When you breathe in and out, every few seconds of every single day, about 20 percent of what you inhale is oxygen. And while oxygen is essential to life, it can also wreak havoc on your cells. I won't bore you with an in-depth biochemistry lesson, but it's important to remember that every healthy cell in your body has molecules with a balanced composition of protons, electrons, and neutrons. When oxygen is processed throughout your body (not just in and out of your lungs, but everywhere), it creates free radicals. Free radicals are molecules that are not balanced, as they contain unpaired electrons. They have a single unbalanced electron orbiting the atom, rather than a balanced pair of electrons. Though the body can handle some free radicals—and in fact, needs *some* to sustain life—having too many free radicals in your body causes damage. That's because all free radicals want to do is find a molecule with paired electrons, so they can steal an electron and have a complete pair. When this happens in your body—as it does every moment you're alive—the formerly complete molecule becomes damaged. This in itself would be fine, because your cells have a crew of molecules to repair the damage, but if the crew is overwhelmed—which it often is—the injury remains unrepaired and starts harming other parts of the cell.

The best way to describe the process of oxidation, in a completely unscientific way, is to compare it to ants on a picnic table set for a party. An ant or two on the picnic table isn't so bad—you can take care of the problem if you notice it early enough. But just as having hundreds or thousands of ants on the table eating away at the foods you've just set up for your guests will ruin a party, excess free radicals can overwhelm the mechanisms your cells have of protecting themselves.

And just as ants are not the only pests that can ruin your picnic, free radicals are not the only oxidants that can ruin your cells. Any chemical that steals electrons is an oxidant. In addition to free radicals and oxygen ions, peroxides (such as hydrogen peroxide) are oxidants. Oxidants come from many sources, from outside your body as well as within your body. Air pollutants from car exhaust or cigarette smoke contains oxidants. Pesticides and herbicides on your foods contain oxidants. Even foods themselves, when they are cooked or processed, can contain oxidants. For example, potatoes are naturally loaded with antioxidants, but deep-frying potatoes into french fries causes them to be loaded with free radicals. The same thing happens with processed foods exposed to excess oxygen, heat, and chemicals while they are being made. Some oxidants cause your foods to turn rancid in taste, but many others remain hidden. Even the medicines we take sometimes contain or even *are* oxidants. Ultraviolet radiation from sun exposure creates oxidants inside cells. And metals, which we'll talk about later in this chapter, can be oxidants too. What can be done?

HOW OXIDANTS CAUSE DAMAGE

What causes damage to your body is not the oxidants themselves, but their actions in stealing electrons. This is because these electrons are taken from the proteins your cells need to stay healthy and from the lipids your cells need to form their cell membrane (their outer coat). When oxidants decide to take over DNA, there's big trouble because that process of DNA damage may lead to disease, cancer, and excess aging. (We'll talk more about DNA in chapter 4.)

For our purposes, it's more important to know how the presence of oxidants in the body can speed up the progress of degenerative conditions that affect the eye, including glaucoma, cataracts, retinitis pigmentosa, and macular degeneration. The eye is exposed to a lot of oxygen, and oxidation, every day. The highest blood flow per cubic millimeter of anywhere in the body is in the eye, right behind the retina. And the most active brain cells of the whole body are those located in the retina. Add in intense light exposure from normal everyday life and you have a lot of oxidation that occurs in the back of the eye every day. Having a lot of oxidants in your body can also accelerate other aspects of the aging process, such as the natural deterioration of your vision in general, as well as increase inflammation (which we'll talk about in chapter 2), and cause damage to blood vessels (which we'll talk about in chapter 3).

So, is there anything you can do to stop the pesky oxidants from taking over? Definitely. You can slow or even dramatically decrease the chain reaction of oxidants inside your body, simply by eating more antioxidants.

Antioxidants are a group of nutrients and vitamins that help protect cells from free radicals. Every antioxidant, whether it's vitamin C or lutein, has electrons to spare so that when an oxidant steals electrons from an antioxidant, it is neutralized and cannot steal any more electrons from any other cells. And neutralized molecules are exactly that—neutral. The process of oxidation stops there. Better yet, some antioxidants—like alpha-lipoic acid—won't stop with just one electron-donating reaction—they engage in multiple electron-donating reactions or they recruit and recycle other oxidants, thus protecting you much further.

You've probably heard commercials for different food products—fruit-flavored yogurt, or perhaps orange juice—touting their antioxidant properties. And while I'm sure those products have benefit, the single best way to "eat your antioxidants" is to eat the natural food wherein the antioxidants exist.

A great example of how this works in real life is called "The French Paradox." You may have heard of this before; it was the idea behind the book, *French Women Don't Get Fat*. A study several years ago discovered that despite the fact that people in various regions of France ate a very high-fat, high-carbohydrate diet (lots of cheese and bread), which should have been associated with a high heart disease risk and rate, their actual rates and risk levels were really low. When scientists examined their diet more closely, they realized that the French were consuming a lot of powerful antioxidants in the form of fruits and vegetables as well as grape- and berry-derived juices, with relatively little processed foods. The overwhelming conclusion from scientists was that the good nutrients in the diet (particularly, bioflavonoids) were out-powering the fatty foods, making those French people, as a whole, healthier than expected.

THE ROLE OF BIOFLAVONOIDS

Bioflavonoids are a group of thousands of nutrients found in plant foods. We actually don't need to eat bioflavonoids for our bodies or cells to function, but we get a lot of benefits when we do: These nutrients are not only antioxidants, but are anti-cancer, anti-infectious (i.e., they boost your immunity, which we'll also discuss in chapter 2), anti-allergy, and anti-inflammatory. And pretty delicious if you ask me: coffee, tea, chocolate (dark, without the sugar and fat), and berries are high in bioflavonoids. Bioflavonoids are also found in red peppers, sweet peppers, citrus fruit, garlic, spinach, and apples. That's why "an apple a day keeps the doctor away," but it's smart to eat more than just apples, because our bodies need more antioxidants than one apple a day provides.

In binding metals, bioflavonoids prevent them from causing oxidation within your body. You may be thinking, I have metals in my body? Yes, you do—everyone does. And having some metal is good for you, just like having some vitamins and some bacteria. Think of iron, for example. But unfortunately, science has shown that most of us come into contact with far too much metal in our environment.

Here's a good example of how easily we can encounter metal in everyday life. Several years ago, my son did a science project for school, where he bought coffee mugs from common big-box retailers and tested each using a home lead test kit. He found that every mug made in China contained lead on its surface even after washing, while the mugs made in the United States and Italy did not. It's so easy to accidentally ingest a metal as dangerous as lead—and it happens all the time.

Metals are in our air, our drinking water, our soil, and in our food, even in medications. In fact, some vitamin and fish oil pills have metals, which can stem from their sources or their manufacturing. In her Pulitzer Prize–winning book *Behind the Beautiful Forevers,* author Katherine Boo shares a story about how the poor living in slums near the Mumbai airport sell fish caught from sewage-polluted streams to manufacturers of fish oil; this is but one example of how supplements from around the world easily become tainted. Metals also leach into our food supply from the diet of farm animals or from processing meats, as shown in many documentaries concerning the source of animal products in the United States and elsewhere.

Unfortunately, these are just a few of the ways we can unknowingly come into contact with toxic metals. But there are also a few targeted ways to avoid known sources of ingested metals:

1. **Avoid processed foods.** The more your meal is processed, the more machines your food has come into physical contact with. The more machines your food touches, the more likely

that metals from those machines have leached into it. If you eat unprocessed food, the chance of it coming into contact with metals is minimal at best. And don't forget about all those other oxidants we discussed earlier that go into processed foods. If possible, go organic, to avoid herbicides and pesticides that can contain toxins and metals such as arsenic.

2. **Avoid air pollution.** From cigarette smoke and car exhaust, to other gas fumes, these pollutants contain toxic metals that, once inhaled, may be immensely hard to get out of your body. Even as you walk around an idling car or a person smoking outside a building, simply increasing your distance can help minimize your contact. Also, be sure to jog or bike away from busy roadways if you can.

3. **Avoid toxic metals at home.** Beyond lead paint, art supplies can contain mercury; plastics (such as vinyl) that are used to make lunchboxes, toys, and furniture can contain lead and toxins; some costume jewelry and even children's jewelry can contain toxic metals including lead and cadmium; and dishware can contain lead. Test items in your home for lead. A home test kit like my son used is easy to buy. Pay attention to where the things you buy are made and avoid buying products made in countries whose products test positive for lead in your home today. While you can't go back in time and mitigate past risk, you can make healthier choices for your family.

THE ROLE OF PHYTIC ACID

Luckily, nature—in the form of nutrition—helps us minimize the effects of metals within our bodies, taking them out of action by

binding the metals, thereby preventing oxidation. A major nuent that plays this role in your body is phytic acid, found in bea
(including soybean tofu, lentils, navy beans, white beans, and chickpeas), grains (whole wheat bread, whole wheat pasta, and wild rice),
vegetables (spinach, carrots, olives, and beets) and even seeds and
nuts (Brazil nuts, almonds, and walnuts). A bit of a super-nutrient,
phytic acid not only binds and removes metals like aluminum, cadmium, lead, and mercury from your body, but it also has been shown
to prevent the cell proliferation that leads to cancer. Phytic acid also
has a role in maintaining the body's messengers that send signals
between cells, such as the signals that help clean up debris from the
retina (we'll talk more about this harmful debris in chapter 7).

However, you must be careful about incorporating the right
amount of phytic acid in your diet, because it is also a strong binder
of good metals, such as iron. Iron is essential for transporting oxygen into your blood cells, so having too much phytic acid binds too
much iron and can lead to an iron deficiency (commonly known as
anemia). Some of the symptoms of anemia include fatigue, shortness of breath, increased heart rate, pale skin, and brittle nails.

It's important to note that, like iron, not all metals are bad. Some
actually help fight oxidation by supporting antioxidant enzymes;
many help our bodies function in other ways. But you always have to
be careful about how much of the good metals you ingest, because
taking too much can also lead to problems.

THE GOOD METALS

You might be wondering, what makes a metal "good" or "bad"? At
a molecular level there are a lot of reasons, but ultimately this designation is determined by how the metal helps your body function
better or worse—for example how the iron (used in constructing a
skyscraper) can help your blood bring oxygen to the retina or the

naking the walls of your soda can) may be part
ess that eventually leads to macular degenera-
both metals listed in this section are not only
pically help antioxidants do their job in finding
ualizing those pesky free radicals discussed earlier. If you
want to slow oxidation, and thereby slow aging and its correspond-
ing physical ailments, these are the nutrients (and foods) to eat:

1. **Manganese:** This metal plays a central role in a powerful
   antioxidant enzyme—called manganese superoxide dis-
   mutase—that works in mitochondria (the power plants
   of your cells). It helps many other enzymes, such as those
   that create the scaffolding of the optic nerve and the eye
   filtration site (we'll talk more about these in chapter 8 on
   glaucoma), prevent diabetes, coat nerve fibers, and support
   normal blood clotting mechanisms. Manganese is found
   in pine nuts, hazelnuts, and pecans as well as wheat bread,
   pineapple, and coconut. It's best ingested in combination
   with leafy greens, making a kale salad with pine nuts a perfect way to add manganese to your diet.

2. **Magnesium:** This metal is a great nutrient for many reasons: first and foremost, it activates almost all the enzyme
   reactions involved in the creation of the universal energy
   packet—called ATP—of all your cells. They need magnesium to make energy! Magnesium is also important for
   hundreds of enzymes and for the body's ability to make proteins. Not only does it prevent oxidation, it also helps your
   muscles relax, your blood vessels regulate flow (we'll learn
   more about this in chapter 7), and more specifically to the
   eye it helps the lens maintain its clarity and prevents corneal
   infections and dry eye. Beans, including black beans, lima

beans, and kidney beans, contain a lot of magnesium, as does spinach, sole, and shrimp.

YOUR ANTIOXIDANT ARMY

As an eye surgeon, I see what oxidation does to your eyes firsthand. Although free radicals and oxidants cause damage to your entire body, oxidants truly wreak havoc on the eye—because it has the highest blood flow per cubic millimeter of anywhere in the body, because it has the most metabolically active cells, because it has amazingly transparent tissue, among other unique and amazing features about the eye we've already learned. This means that in addition to having oxidants of its own (which reside in the components of the eye), free radicals come visiting from other parts of the body looking for cells to attack—making the eye more susceptible to damage.

The body does know to send more antioxidants and protective nutrients to the eye, but it's always helpful to provide more boots on the ground. There are three important antioxidant soldiers you can send in to help fight your body's war on oxidation: sulforaphane, glutathione, and alpha-lipoic acid.

The first soldier, sulforaphane, is a plant chemical that has been shown to protect the whole eye against oxidation. But it's not an antioxidant soldier itself. Rather it acts like a military commander who recruits a team of antioxidants and gears them up for action. Its recruits are antioxidant enzymes called "phase 2" enzymes, which go into the battlefield. Sulforaphane also activates many antioxidants inside your body and, when paired up with glutathione, becomes incredibly effective. It also has other helpful properties, including anti-inflammatory and anti-cancer actions.

The best source for sulforaphane is baby broccoli sprouts (which are harvested and eaten within a few days of sprouting), though broccoli spears, brussels sprouts, and red cabbage are also good sources. Sulforaphane's very sharp, bitter taste acts as a protective agent for the plant it comes from. Animals stay away because they don't like the taste, and it's a natural pesticide. This may be why it's primarily found in baby broccoli sprouts and the spears of broccoli but not the "tree," or floret part of adult broccoli that humans and animals prefer.

The second soldier to include in your antioxidant army is sulforaphane's best buddy, glutathione. Composed of three amino acids linked together, glutathione protects the retina, macula, and the cornea from damage by powerfully neutralizing some of the most damaging oxidants and also by helping other enzymes and antioxidants such as vitamin E do their work, and by recycling other antioxidants, such as vitamin C. One of the most glutathione-rich foods is asparagus, and it can also be found in ground beef, steak, chicken liver, walnuts, and spinach. Eating your soldiers is a great excuse for ordering beef and vegetable stir-fry—I like to order a healthy preparation from my local kosher Chinese restaurant: a steamed version, sauce on the side, with brown steamed rice!

Last but not least, the third soldier in your army is alpha-lipoic acid. Nicknamed the "Antioxidant of Antioxidants," this vitamin-like nutrient is so potent and powerful it should be ranked as a colonel. Once it fights off one oxidant by donating an electron for the oxidant to steal, alpha-lipoic acid transforms into an even more potent version of itself (called dihydrolipoic acid), which is at least twenty to thirty times more powerful than the original. It can restore antioxidant properties to other antioxidants that become "used-up" after having already stopped an oxidant (that's why it is the "Antioxidant of Antioxidants"). It also can bind metals to prevent them from acting as oxidants. It lowers oxidative stress in the blood, an important preventative measure against damage in the retina and the eye as a whole. Found in brussels sprouts, tomatoes, peas, steak, and spinach, alpha-lipoic acid is a powerful antioxidant everyone should include in their diet.

But before you go shopping, listen to the following cautionary tale.

WHEN TOO MUCH OF A GOOD THING CAN BE DOWNRIGHT HARMFUL

We all know some people who simply can't resist jumping on the latest "discovery" heralded on the evening news, in a newspaper headline, or simply on a package of juice—making it their primary tool in improving a condition or their overall health. And though most of the time we're all doing our best to stay informed, sometimes we don't know the whole story.

For instance, I had a patient, who I'll call Jane, come to my office in tears. Jane flew in to see me from across the country after multiple other doctors couldn't figure out why her vision was increasingly blurry. Though Jane could see well enough to drive and get around her house, she couldn't read or order off a restaurant menu.

One of the doctors she had previously visited did see some swelling in her retina but couldn't figure out why. When I sat down with her and examined her eyes, I also asked about supplements, since many people take vitamins that negatively interact with the function of the eye. Jane said she was taking a stress-relief formula of vitamin B, which contained about 100 milligrams each of vitamin B1, B2, B3, and B6 along with 100 micrograms of B12. The capsule was supposed to be taken once a day, but Jane thought her stress levels warranted taking two a day. (Jane is the assistant to a very demanding executive.) She also told me that she had frequent headaches, had been vomiting frequently, and had lost a pretty substantial amount of weight since she had started taking the vitamin supplement. After she said that, I knew that the supplement was her problem.

The excess vitamin B6 caused the headaches and weight loss. And the vitamin B3 she was taking (about 200 milligrams a day) caused the swelling in her retina that made her vision blurry. Typically, a person would have to consume 1,500 milligrams a day for the retina to swell, but there are many exceptions to what clinicians and doctors consider "standards." Jane had been taking her stress-relief formula for a very long time, about five to ten years.

I asked Jane to stop taking the supplement, and when she came to visit me for a follow-up six weeks later, I saw an entirely different person. Not only was her vision back to normal, but her headaches and vomiting had stopped and she was slowly returning to a healthy weight. Ironically, she was much less stressed, even though her boss was the same tough person as before.

There are two lessons I want to share from Jane's story. First, not all "results" or "discoveries" you hear on the news work for everyone. Vitamin B complex can help relieve stress, but for some people like Jane, even a seemingly small excess amount can cause more harm than good.

And second, this is a good example of why I recommend that people eat natural vitamin-rich foods rather than using supplements or eating enriched, processed foods. Numerous clinical studies, as well as anecdotal evidence from my practice and patients like Jane, suggest that antioxidant vitamins are often much less effective when removed from their natural food sources. In fact, some nutrients can actually cause *more* oxidative damage if people accidentally ingest too much of certain vitamins or nutrients by mistake. Here are three vitamins to watch out for, because too much of a good thing can result in excess oxidation and damage:

1. **Vitamin C:** Top sources to include in your diet are peppers, broccoli, strawberries, mangoes, and oranges. The chance that you'll get truly sick from having too much vitamin C is

low, though this vitamin, particularly if taken as pills, will give you a stomachache if you eat too much. We often talk about vitamin C protecting against the common cold, but interestingly there is very little scientific evidence to prove that. But there *is* a lot of scientific evidence—sixteen medical studies—proving that vitamin C protects against cataracts. With all this data supporting vitamin C's protective effects against cataracts, then shouldn't we be munching down a lot of vitamin C pills? Well, a recent study of nearly twenty-five thousand women showed vitamin C actually *increased* the risk of cataracts—going against everything we've learned. Why? Because in this study the vitamin C was taken without the appropriate balance of antioxidants. The excess vitamin C—without any other antioxidants to balance it—itself becomes oxidized into a chemical called dehydroascorbate, causing sugars to stick to the proteins of the lens, damaging the proteins, and reducing the transparency of the lens—causing cataracts (we'll talk more about cataracts in chapter 9), another example of how too much of a good thing can be bad, particularly if not balanced with other good nutrients.

2. **Vitamin E:** Top sources to include in your diet are almonds, seafood, spinach, asparagus, and kiwis. Vitamin E is a powerful antioxidant that may help protect the eye from many conditions, ranging from cataracts to glaucoma. But like many vitamins, it can cause nausea and stomachaches if you eat too much. More important, high amounts increase the risk of bleeding inside the body and can trigger more problems, such as strokes (from bleeding in the brain). When taken in excess, vitamin E is an oxidant itself and blocks the action of other antioxidants, such as vitamin A. In excess, it can prevent your body from absorbing vitamin A, D, and

K. In chapter 5, we'll talk more about the dangers of vitamin E and you'll hear the story of Sharon—who had a toxic
buildup of vitamin A caused by excess vitamin E.

3. **Vitamin B2:** Found in feta cheese, yogurt, eggs, and mushrooms, vitamin B2 will act like an oxidant and directly affect
the lens of the eye and the retina if taken in excess. Vitamin
B2 is known as a "cellular photosensitizer." In other words,
in the presence of light, vitamin B2 can absorb light and
become "excited." By becoming energetically excited, it
pulls in electrons and creates oxidants.

Nutrition is a tricky balance to strike: You want to eat enough, so
your body has the tools and soldiers it needs to fight the war against
aging, oxidation, and other types of damage, but if you go too far,
you might end up aiding the other side. Go for the natural sources
of vitamin C, E, and B2, and you should be in good shape—you'll
get enough without going over, and you'll get many other nutrients
to balance these.

Nowhere else in your diet is that balance closer than when it
comes to eating minerals, such as the metals iron and zinc. You
absolutely need them to help your body and eyes be healthy, but
eating more than what your body should have can greatly *increase*
the speed and rate of oxidation.

Metals to Limit in Your Diet

Despite essential benefits of metals, they can be harmful in high
amounts.

Copper: Though copper does a lot of wonderful things—like
helping antioxidants do their job, assisting in regulating blood flow
and in iron transportation, protecting against damage from sunlight by forming light-absorbing pigment granules, and helping to

form collagen for areas of your eye like the cornea, retina, and optic nerve—high consumption of copper causes oxidation and has been linked to vision-related disease. Beef liver is quite high in copper; other top sources that will give you healthy amounts include nuts, avocados, lobster, and crab.

Zinc: You may be familiar with this metal's cold-fighting abilities (zinc has been shown to boost immunity); it also assists antioxidant processes, protects against sunlight damage, and helps our genes function properly. But at high concentrations in the body, zinc *causes* oxidation and damages neurons by blocking their growth signals. Be wary of too much zinc. Oysters are extremely high in zinc, but lentils and beans, nuts, cheeses, meats, and chocolate will give you healthy amounts as long as you don't gorge. Because of how zinc and copper compete with each other for absorption in the gut, you will want to balance the two with a ratio of tenfold zinc to onefold copper, otherwise you'll throw off your cholesterol levels and you may end up with an excess or a deficiency of copper or zinc—for example, a deficiency of copper can cause anemia, increased infections, and a variety of eye diseases. Think of how you use small portions of cheese or avocado to accent a salad, whereas a bean burrito might be a main course. Many natural foods, such as nuts, that have copper and zinc are often properly balanced, while supplement pills may be imbalanced.

Iron: We should walk a nutritional tightrope with iron—you absolutely need iron to carry oxygen in your blood and prevent anemia. In chapter 3, we'll talk more about all its numerous essential benefits. However, iron is a metal that steals electrons—so, it is an oxidant. When eating a healthy balanced diet (we'll learn about that in Part III), it is hard to overdose on iron, and you'll get enough antioxidants to balance its oxidant effects. Some people need iron pills to supplement their diet and prevent anemia, but these sometimes have unintended problems. Good natural sources of iron are nuts, beef, spinach, beans, and tofu.

Selenium: This metal does a lot—it assists enzymes throughout your body, some of which are antioxidants. It also helps recycle vitamin C, protects the eye from oxidative damage, and can minimize the risk of developing macular degeneration and cataracts. It even boosts immunity. Along with vitamin B2 and vitamin E, it creates the enzyme that produces glutathione. But don't let selenium's assets fool you: it's still highly toxic—it can cause hair loss, brittle nails, even heart attacks and kidney failure. A previous study stunned the medical community when it showed that a seemingly mild (perhaps only somewhat high) dose of selenium—200 micrograms per day as opposed to my often suggested 50 to 100 micrograms per day—doubled the risk of developing glaucoma! Your body needs so small of a dose that it's easy to go overboard. Brazil nuts have the most selenium of any food; eating just a handful can put your body over its limit. However, good amounts of selenium are found in a regular serving of eggs, steak, and seafood.

Oxidation has a lot to do with aging. While we haven't yet found the fountain of youth—and don't fully understand the process of aging—good nutrition and eating a lot of antioxidant foods have been shown to slow down the effects of aging. In addition, as we age our metabolism slows and we eat less, and so we have lower intake of nutrients. Furthermore, our digestive system becomes less efficient at absorbing the nutrients, leaving us with a relative paucity in many of them. Thus, good nutritional intake becomes even more important as we age. In the upcoming chapters, as we learn about other nutrients and about mechanisms of various eye diseases, you'll see how there is a lot of overlap with vision problems and oxidation.

SUMMARY 1: THE POWER OF OXYGEN

Oxidant—a chemical that steals electrons.

Oxygen creates free radicals—which are one type of oxidant.

Many sources of oxidants: pollutants, pesticides, herbicides, cooked foods, processed foods, some medicines, metals, and others.

Avoid processed foods, air pollution, and toxic metals at home.

Oxidation causes damage to proteins, lipids, and DNA.

Antioxidants have extra electrons to spare so they can "neutralize" oxidants.

Important nutrients from chapter 1:
- Bioflavonoids—nutrients from plant foods.
- Phytic acid—binds and removes metals.
- Manganese—a "good" metal and powerful antioxidant.
- Magnesium—a "good" metal that helps many enzymes.
- Sulforaphane—recruits antioxidants.
- Glutathione—strong antioxidant and recycles other antioxidants.
- Alpha-lipoic acid—the antioxidant of antioxidants.

Too much of a good thing can be a bad thing: too much vitamin C, vitamin E, or vitamin B2 can *cause* oxidation.

Metals that you need, but you shouldn't consume too much of: copper, zinc, iron, and selenium.

CHAPTER 2

FIGHTING INFLAMMATION

There is a saying in medicine that inflammation is the root cause of every single disease. Inflammation is indeed powerful and can cause a wide array of damage to our bodies. However, the body is a complex organism and there is often considerable overlap between the various mechanisms of health disorders. This is why simple answers—such as the saying above—often fail to take into consideration the complexity of the situation. The science of medicine clearly identifies various other mechanisms—or root causes of illnesses—such as those we are examining in this book. That said, the power of inflammation is certainly a big factor in how health disorders develop and progress.

The word "inflammation" comes from the Latin "to set afire, to ignite" (*in flammo,* or in flame), and so we think of it as a bad thing. It is true; inflammation can often damage the body. However, inflammation is also very helpful to the body in many circumstances, particularly in fighting off infections. Yes, inflammation produces those terrible fevers we get when we're sick, but perhaps the fever is helpful in getting rid of the inciting bug by increasing the body's ability to attack it.

INFLAMMATION TO START THE HEALING PROCESS

Maybe inflammation is not the root cause of every disease, but it certainly plays a role in a wide array of conditions. In the eye, inflammation can indeed be harmful and has been shown to play a role in every single condition we talk about in Part II of this book. Having the proper immune response, however, may protect your eyesight.

Common expressions of inflammation in our bodies include infections, allergies, and responses to physical injuries and burns, as well as a whole host of common conditions such as asthma, bronchitis, sinusitis, gastritis, laryngitis, and arthritis. There are even times when the body is fooled into believing that the intruder is itself, and so it starts attacking itself (auto-immune disease).

While inflammation can cause a variety of symptoms from fevers and chills to redness and swelling to pain, some inflammation is painless and without any symptoms. Most notably, though, inflammation can cause damage. But how? And why would it do so?

Let's talk about how inflammation works on a cellular and molecular level.

AN ARMY OF THUGS OR PRECISION WARRIORS?

Inflammation is when the body recruits its army of white blood cells, antibodies, and specialized chemicals to attack an intruder—whether the intruder is alive like a bug or inanimate like a noxious chemical—and then start the body's healing process. Well that sounds wonderful: getting rid of the bad guys, and then starting the *healing*!

The white blood cells, antibodies, and specialized chemicals perform a series of actions: First they recruit more white blood cells, antibodies, and specialized chemicals by calling out to their colleagues or by throwing out flares and other signals. By increasing the blood flow to the area where the intruders are, they can more easily deliver these additional recruits. But they also make blood vessels leaky, so that the white blood cells, antibodies, and specialized chemicals can exit the blood vessel highway and get to the place they need to go. Inflammation also initiates blood clotting and anti-clotting mechanisms when needed. And the army attacks, ingests, destroys, and removes intruders—sometimes by physically eating them up and other times by shooting out toxic chemicals or a combination of these approaches.

Although this is a gross oversimplification of the process of inflammation, you can see the body has quite a large arsenal at its disposal, often with precision capability. However, no war is pleasant and even precision strikes have collateral damage to innocent people and the lands in which they live. The body's no exception, as its attack on intruders and noxious chemicals can result in much damage to the surrounding tissue and organs where the attack is being mounted, causing them to malfunction or even stop working, through varied mechanisms such as leaking fluid, pus accumulation, scarring, and death of tissue.

To make things even more complicated, inflammation can be localized or occur throughout the whole body. It can start suddenly and end just as suddenly, or it can drag on for months, years, and decades.

INFLAMMATION IN THE EYE

In the eye, inflammation can cause or exacerbate macular degeneration, retinitis pigmentosa, diabetic retinopathy, glaucoma, cataracts, and dry eye. Macular degeneration (see chapter 5) is a disorder in which debris starts to accumulate beneath the retina, ultimately causing damage that decreases vision. It's not all about the debris, though. It seems to be caused by a combination of environmental insults with genetic predispositions. Science is just now starting to discover the genes that are the risk factors involved in various forms of macular degeneration. And guess what? Four of the first six genes that have been discovered are involved in inflammation. It's worth mentioning these first genes by name, because of their historical significance in the understanding of macular degeneration: complement factor H (CFH or Factor H), complement factor B (CFB), complement component 2 (C2), and chemokine ligand 1 (CX3CL1). These genes all code for either a signaling protein or assistant proteins that "complement" the inflammation process. The other two genes are involved in the process of removal of debris—or drusen—which we'll learn about in chapter 5. As we find more genes involved, many continue to be ones involved in inflammation.

A defect in a gene involved in inflammation causes that gene to function improperly—what the body is supposed to accomplish may not happen, and damage to tissue—whether the damage is large scale or microscopic—is likely to occur. Methods of damage with inflammation—the leaking of fluid, pus accumulation, scarring, and death of tissue—play various roles in a tremendously wide variety of eye conditions.

TREATMENT FOR INFLAMMATION

So how do we treat inflammation? The short answer is through medications such as:

- aspirin and aspirin-like products, including over-the-counter ibuprofen and naproxen

- steroids, technically what are called corticosteroids, such as cortisone

- chemotherapy types of medicines that often brutally and indiscriminately attack the inflammation

- antibody medications; biological agents that attack the inflammation by binding to them in the same way that the body's own antibodies attack perceived intruders.

But often, in the eye conditions we discuss in this book, inflammation is either an ongoing or a low-grade, subtle process. Treating inflammation in the eye by taking these medications by mouth may be tough on the whole body—in addition to blocking the unwanted inflammation they can block the good inflammation necessary to protect ourselves and thus leave us vulnerable to attack from other intruders and noxious chemicals—and they can cause a lot of unwanted side effects. Even aspirin can cause heartburn and stomach ulcers, bleeding complications, electrolyte imbalances, and even in rare cases serious liver damage—and these are considered less serious side effects when compared to those of steroids and the biological agents. This is why, many times, we can't take these medicines long-term.

So what alternatives do we have to these medications?

NUTRITION TO BALANCE AND CONTROL INFLAMMATION

Plants have numerous ways to help them ward off intruders, such as a rose's sharp thorns to make it unappetizing, or a tree's sticky sap (called resin) that traps insects and even small amphibians, to keep them from boring into its core. Even the itchy chemical produced by the poison ivy plant . . . we all know to avoid that! The surfaces of some plants also have deterrent pungent smells, some remarkably complex: When a cabbage leaf is cut on a live plant—and a juicy bite is taken—it emits a scent to which nearby cabbage plants respond and together the cabbages in the cabbage patch emit a toxin to deter the predator.

For thousands of years, humans have been using plants to help treat our ailments. Aspirin was initially isolated from a chemical in the bark of the willow tree, the same chemical the tree uses to deter many insects and even larger animals like deer and moose, a chemical that can be deadly to these animals.

Phytochemicals (*phyto* meaning plant in Greek) are found in plants that affect the biological activity of animals and may be beneficial for humans in helping decrease blood pressure, reducing the risk of cancer, and preventing heart disease and diabetes. What follows is an overview of some important phytochemicals—in Part II we'll talk about phytochemicals useful for specific eye conditions.

Bioflavonoids, some of our favorite antioxidants from chapter 1, are very important anti-inflammatory agents. The body has natural inflammatory pathways—all those series of actions that the white blood cells, antibodies, and specialized chemicals perform. Bioflavonoids jump in the middle and stop them, often by blocking specific enzymes needed to either start up these processes or keep them going.

Some of the phytochemicals are *phytoalexins*, substances produced in response to an intruder that help us ward off viral or bacterial infections or help our antioxidant defense mechanisms. Other phytochemicals are *phytoanticipins*, substances produced in the day-to-day protective mechanisms of healthy plants. Given the thousands of different bioflavonoids, they are sure to help you throughout life.

Quercetin, for example, is one of the most active bioflavonoids with many functions. As with other bioflavonoids, your body doesn't need quercetin to function, but it is quite helpful in controlling inflammation and helping the body respond to such diseases as diabetes (for more on this, see chapter 7). It can block some of the enzymes needed to start inflammation and keep it going. It can act as an antihistamine, decreasing allergic reactions (histamines are one of those specialized chemicals involved in the process of creating inflammation in allergic responses). Quercetin can control inflammation in other ways as well. Sometimes in inflammation, white blood cells get stuck to other tissue, such as the walls of blood vessels—when this happens, they start waging their battle right where they're stuck, but maybe that's not where they are needed.

Quercetin comes to the rescue to "unstick" them by decreasing their ability to adhere to these sites. In addition, quercetin itself can attack viruses and inhibit the activity of viruses.

Quercetin is present in a wide variety of fruits and vegetables. Top sources include hot chile peppers, red onions, and bee pollen—the bees' collection of some of the best nutrients from plants. It is also found in unsweetened cocoa powder, raw cranberries and lingonberries, onions, kale, cilantro, broccoli, and okra.

Back in 1990, President George H. W. Bush famously confessed to hate broccoli: "I haven't liked it since I was a little kid and my mother made me eat it. [Now] I'm President of the United States, and I'm not going to eat any more broccoli!" Later, President Barack Obama claimed that broccoli is his favorite food, out of any food in the whole world. But why is it that broccoli is so important? It turns out that broccoli contains a biologically active compound called diindolylmethane—also called DIM—known to have strong anti-cancer activity. For the eye, it alters expression of genes to boost immune defense but yet control inflammation. DIM is found in the "cruciferous" vegetables—so called because the petals of their flowers form a cross—including broccoli, cauliflower, brussels sprouts, cabbage, kale, bok choy, and watercress. You may recall that some of these vegetables are also very high in the potent antioxidant sulforaphane that we learned about in chapter 1. So having broccoli at the top of your list of favorite foods is certainly a good thing.

And with all the talk about how plants ward off intruders, no discussion can be complete without mentioning mushrooms. Some mushrooms are deadly poisonous, perhaps to kill off hungry predators or to help them dig their "roots" into trees. One group of what we term as healthy mushrooms, called *agaricus*—which includes the white button mushroom often seen on pizza as well as the large portobello mushroom—also contains a compound called lectin.

Lectins are often harmful to humans, causing immune responses and allergies. This is why we cook foods such as beans and potatoes—to deactivate these lectins! However, some lectins may be beneficial, as they stick to certain sugar-proteins on the surface of inflammatory cells and prevent these cells from proliferating. This activity from the agaricus lectin (agartine), found in mushrooms, is believed to control inflammation and perhaps can even inhibit scar tissue formation. Just be careful and don't overdo it—some mushrooms are high in selenium, and you don't want too much selenium.

If you purchase a supplement (as in a pill) that has a phytochemical nutrient in it, keep in mind that the FDA does not require the manufacturer to prove that the phytochemical nutrient is either effective or even safe—as long as they do not claim it cures or treats any medical condition. Just because there's no warning label on these pills doesn't mean you do not need to be careful about what they contain. True, fruits and vegetables also don't come with any warning label. The difference is that humans have had thousands of years of experience with fruits and vegetables—we know that apples are safe but don't eat the apple seeds. We may not know that apple seeds are full of a chemical called amygdalin that is converted by our gut enzymes into cyanide—we just know from our ancestors that it's a bad idea to eat them. So rather than blindly ingesting supplements that may contain one or a few of the many known bioflavonoids—and miss many others that we don't yet even know about—go for the natural sources of nutrients.

You'll find the theme of inflammation appears repeatedly throughout this book, and we'll see that more than just phytochemicals can help battle against it: we'll learn about garlic in chapter 8, curry spice in chapter 6, omega-3 and omega-6 oils in chapters 6 and 10, and taurine, boron, and resveratrol in chapter 7.

SUMMARY 2: FIGHTING INFLAMMATION

Inflammation is a body's response to infections, allergens, physical injuries and burns, and other ailments.

Inflammation occurs when the body recruits white blood cells, antibodies, and/or specialized chemicals.

Inflammation is necessary to protect the body but can also cause damage—sometimes permanent—to the body.

Treatment for inflammation can come from medications or from good nutrition.

Important nutrients from chapter 2:

- Bioflavonoids—nutrients from plant foods.

- Quercetin—one of the most active bioflavonoids.

- Diindolylmethane—also known as DIM, a powerful nutrient.

- Agaricus—healthful mushrooms that are anti-inflammatory.

CHAPTER 3

OPTIMIZING BLOOD FLOW AND BLOOD VESSELS

Our blood is our life. For isn't that why our hearts beat: to deliver blood throughout our body? Blood delivers oxygen and nutrients and removes toxic wastes, sending it to our kidneys and livers for filtration and detoxification. Blood delivers white blood cells and specialized chemical agents (as discussed in chapter 2) and it also delivers hormones, which are signaling molecules. Blood even regulates our body temperature and pH. There is a whole field of medicine devoted to the study of blood in health and disease called hematology, and every physician appreciates the importance and central role that blood and our blood vessels play in our health and well-being.

As German author and intellectual Johann Wolfgang von Goethe wrote in his famous tragic play *Faust*: "Blood is a very special juice." Blood is actually considered a body tissue, composed of red blood cells and various types of white blood cells, platelets for clotting and fixing blood vessel breaks, and plasma, the fluid in which these cells and platelets swim. Nutrients, proteins, and hormones—as well as the waste products—are mixed into the plasma. Red blood cells are the taxicabs that pick up oxygen from the lungs and deliver it to our tissues; they have an iron-rich protein called hemoglobin inside of them that grabs the oxygen and takes it along for the ride. Red blood cells live for about four months before degenerating and being replaced by new ones.

Full-sized adults have about a gallon-and-a-quarter to a gallon-and-a-half of blood within their bodies. By weight that's about ten pounds of blood. The heart—which beats one hundred thousand times each day—has the incredible task of pumping out about twenty-five hundred gallons of blood every day, through the sixty thousand miles or so of blood vessels within the body. That's enough miles of blood vessels to encircle the Earth (at its equator) more than twice!

When your blood is in trouble, your eyesight may be able to give you clues. This was the case with a thirty-something-year-old semi-professional golfer we'll call Ben. He came to see me complaining of an intermittent white-out of his vision about once or twice every week. Everything he saw in the world around him would suddenly fade away and stay white for a few minutes and then return to normal. It had been going on for a few months and happened during exertion on the golf course at times. The first time he came and saw me, I said, "Ben, let's get some blood tests and get you over to a cardiologist . . . There's an issue getting blood up from your heart." Upon further questioning, Ben had admitted to feeling more tired than usual and having pains in his legs and arms, which he attributed to his rigorous golf schedule. In examining his eyes, I found no abnormalities whatsoever; nevertheless, his story made it apparent to me that—among the list of possible causes—decreased blood supply was causing these symptoms we call "amaurosis fugax." A few days later, the combination of the blood tests and the cardiologist's evaluation confirmed the diagnosis: an inflammatory condition of the blood vessels that subsequently improved with medications.

BLOOD, VASCULATURE, AND YOUR EYES

When ophthalmologists look at your eyes with our specialized microscopes, we can actually see red blood cells as they zip through capillaries. It takes only about eight seconds for blood to go from your heart, through your eye, and back to your heart. When it reaches your eye, the blood slows down to drop off oxygen and nutrients and pick up wastes before speeding back to your heart.

Unbeknownst to most people, the eye needs a tremendous amount of blood (and more specifically, the oxygen and nutrients blood carries) to function properly. In fact, the area behind the retina requires the greatest blood flow per cubic milliliter of anywhere in our bodies! Yet at the same time, the only place in the body that receives *no* blood is the human cornea. Rather the cornea relies on a surrounding robust network of vessels to nourish the cells that constantly replace the surface of the cornea, and on the network of vessels within the front of the eye, to create a nutrient-rich fluid inside the eye that bathes the back surface of the cornea. Understanding this, it becomes clear that optimizing the blood flow to your eye can help maintain your vision and proper eye health.

Increased blood flow is among the many health benefits of exercise. A 2014 study of people age forty-three to eighty-six showed that being physically active (as opposed to having a sedentary lifestyle) over a twenty-year period decreased the risk of having poor vision or worse visual impairment by 60 percent!

Restricted blood flow can cause heart disease and heart attacks, kidney damage, stroke, and—when extreme—it can throw the body in a medical state called shock. Conditions such as diabetes or atherosclerosis can cause poor blood flow, resulting in a loss of vision or even blindness. Anemia, a condition caused by a decrease in red blood cells or their ability to carry oxygen, can also have a profound impact on the eyes—sometimes noticeably so, and other times insidiously.

When a young patient—we'll call her Rachel—first came to me, I could not help but notice how thin she was. Lately she had been seeing purple-colored blobs in her vision that jiggled around like Jello. I took a look inside her eyes and saw many bleeds and abnormal blood vessels growing—the kind we see in diabetes—but she didn't have diabetes. She had bulimia, and was very malnourished. Because her body lacked many of the important nutrients it needed, she developed anemia. With a lot of help from a team of providers, we slowly got her back on track, supplementing her diet with specific vitamins. Her anemia has resolved and her vision is back to normal. It's been a long road over many years, but I am proud of how far she's come along.

GOOD NUTRITION CAN HELP

We know that iron is essential for transporting oxygen throughout the body. But you also need copper for iron-transport enzymes and to ensure your body can access the right form of iron it needs. Vitamins B6, B12, and folate activate enzymes needed in the production of hemoglobin. Vitamin A supports the red blood cells as they develop. Vitamins C and E are also involved. It's really a family affair!

Healthy nutrition can do much more than help produce red blood cells that carry oxygen. One building block of proteins—an amino acid—found in many foods is arginine. It can maintain oxygen balance and proper blood flow, particularly in the retina. But more important it is a precursor to the formation of nitric oxide, a signaling molecule that helps blood vessels dilate. Blood vessels can constrict and dilate to adjust how much blood flows through them. When a body tissue requires more blood flow—for any of many reasons such as needing more nutrients or oxygen or white blood cells—then blood vessel dilation helps redirect extra blood to that tissue. In this way, nitric oxide is particularly helpful with regard to diabetes (discussed in depth in chapter 7). You can find arginine in fish, chicken, and steak as well as dairy products. Many nuts such as walnuts and peanuts are also high in arginine, as are the vegetables peas, lima beans, kidney beans, corn, broccoli, and spinach.

Keep in mind, though, that when nitric oxide sits around for too long inside a cell, it can degrade into a toxin called peroxynitrite that causes oxidative damage. So, once again you'll need your antioxidants, of which bioflavonoids are a good choice. Happily, bioflavonoids also improve circulation of the bloodstream. This is because arteries—the blood vessels that deliver to tissue—are surrounded by a lining of muscle, which can squeeze tight to constrict blood vessels and limit blood flow, or can relax to allow blood vessels to dilate. Plenty of research shows that bioflavonoids can relax blood vessel walls, increasing blood flow, and research with animals specifically shows bioflavonoids improve blood flow in the retina, and in doing so can improve the functioning of the retina.

Bioflavonoids offer additional circulatory benefits, such as blocking unhealthy blood clotting particles (platelets) injured by oxidative damage, as well as decreasing excess blood clotting by changing cell signal pathways that trigger platelets. Bioflavonoids can also strengthen the smallest of the blood vessel capillaries and even prevent leakage of fluid, as happens in diabetic fluid buildup, or edema. Consult the appendix for a reminder list of foods rich in bioflavonoids.

CAUTION WITH SOME HERBS AND GREEN LEAVES

In discussing the need to block inflammation and also to block the growth of the abnormal blood vessels, it's important to discuss using herbs for this purpose. It is tempting to regard all leaves and flowers as "natural" and benign, but just as some foods and vitamins can have unwanted side effects, so can plants.

St. John's Wort

The leaves and flower of the herb St. John's wort, for example, can be made into a medicinal compound that may block inflammation and block the growth of the abnormal blood vessels. It sounds like a good choice, right? But let's look at its side effects. St. John's wort is known as a photodynamic or photosensitive agent—when light strikes it, it produces toxic oxidants. So if you eat St. John's wort and then stay in the sun for a while, you'll probably develop a sun rash and sunburn much more easily. Over the long term, it even increases the risk of skin cancer. Livestock that graze and ingest large quantities of St. John's wort often become seriously ill from the sun exposure. And remember that in the eye, light gets focused by our lens to the back of the eye. So with this highly focused light, St. John's wort speeds up cataract formation and retinal disease.

Gingko

This nutrient, extracted from the leaf of the gingko biloba tree, has wonderful anti-inflammatory capabilities and is an antioxidant. It can also block platelet clotting activities and relax muscle around arteries, thereby improving blood flow in the body. In the eye, it has been shown to improve blood flow and remarkably improve the clarity of one's vision, improve color vision, and improve side vision in various eye conditions including diabetes, glaucoma, and macular degeneration. However, in some situations, it can also cause serious and potentially fatal bleeding complications, because of its effect on platelets. When taken with higher amounts of vitamin E or omega-3 oils—two nutrients that can also cause bleeding complications when higher amounts are taken—the risk of bleeding increases. If you're on aspirin or prone to bleed easily, gingko can be seriously problematic.

Vitamin K

While St. John's wort and gingko can increase bleeding by preventing clotting, vitamin K is just the opposite. Vitamin K comes from the German word for clotting: *koagulation* or coagulation in English.

There are three forms of vitamin K: plants make the K1 form called phylloquinone, bacteria make the K2 form called menaquinone, and the K3 form called menadione is synthetic. (Because the synthetic form interferes with the antioxidant glutathione and can accumulate in excess in the bloodstream, the natural forms are better.) Vitamin K activates two important processes: blood clotting and bone building. People who already have cardiovascular risk factors and need their blood to be thinned are told to avoid vitamin K and foods that are high in it (these people may already be on a baby aspirin per day or other agent that blocks blood clotting). For everyone else, vitamin K helps balance the processes and protect the ability of the body to create blood clots when needed. Parsley has the highest concentration of vitamin K of any common vegetable. Other sources are kale, spinach, beet greens, lettuce, broccoli, brussels sprouts, and asparagus.

Laughter Is the Best Medicine

With all this talk about nutrients, perhaps laughter is the best medicine, seriously! A study on some young healthy volunteers watching a fifteen-minute comedy found that a good prolonged laugh increased blood flow by more than 20 percent. There are several hypotheses as to why, including that laughter releases chemicals within the body that relax the muscles that surround arteries. So go ahead and laugh . . . there are many other health benefits to laughter and happiness.

SUMMARY 3: OPTIMIZING BLOOD FLOW AND BLOOD VESSELS

Blood is a body tissue that delivers oxygen, nutrients, inflammatory agents, and hormones. It removes toxic wastes and regulates body temperature and pH.

Blood consists of red blood cells, white blood cells, platelets, nutrients, proteins, and hormones.

Red blood cells have an iron-rich protein called hemoglobin that carries oxygen.

Optimizing blood flow to your eye can help maintain your vision and eye health.

Restricted blood flow can cause damage to the eye.

A family of nutrients is required for healthy blood: iron, copper, folate, and vitamins A, B6, B12, C, and E.

Important nutrients from chapter 3:
- Arginine—an amino acid that maintains oxygen balance and proper blood flow.
- Bioflavonoids—provide additional circulatory benefits.
- St. John's wort—an herb that blocks inflammation and abnormal blood vessel growth.
- Gingko—a plant nutrient that can improve blood flow.
- Vitamin K—supports healthy blood clotting.

Caution with some of these same nutrients:
- St. John's wort—can cause light-induced oxidation.
- Gingko—can cause serious bleeding complications.
- Vitamin K—people with cardiovascular risk factors who need their blood thinned are often told to limit vitamin K intake.

Laughter may be the best medicine—it helps increase blood flow.

CHAPTER 4
FEEDING YOUR GENES AND DNA THROUGHOUT YOUR LIFE

We all have a genetic code written inside us from the day we are born that can dictate, for example, that we will have brown hair instead of blonde or grow tall like Dad instead of being on the short side like Mom. However, what many people don't realize is that we have a whole set of genes that our bodies are constantly turning on and off—like light switches—that affect our health, how our bodies function, and how we feel. We use these genes every moment of every day of our lives, and they can be affected by our behavior: by what we eat and how active we are.

A gene is a unit of heredity in any living organism. And all living organisms depend on genes. A gene consists of stretches of a compound called deoxyribonucleic acid—or DNA for short—that are like an instruction manual for how to build our cells, specifically how to make the proteins that make our cells run.

The language in this book is simple, not nearly as complex as the English language, or Swahili, Hebrew, or Japanese. The alphabet is only four different letters, translated into English as the letters A, C, G, and T. Each word that is created is three letters long—there are no words that are longer or shorter. The book that comes with your body is a long book with about two billion words, arranged in about twenty thousand to twenty-five thousand chapters—each chapter explaining how to make a single gene. That's quite a large book—in fact, if the book was written in English it would be as thick as a stack of about forty thousand copies of the book in your hands, which would stack up about twice the height of the Empire State Building.

But everything's smaller in our cells—if you take all the words from one cell, as they are written in their microscopic print, and line them up end-to-end in a straight line they would stretch about six feet. That's in one cell. If you take all the words from all the thirty-seven trillion or so cells in our bodies, they would form a single-file line stretching for forty billion miles—that's more than ten times farther than the distance from the Sun to Pluto.

Some chapters of the book—genes—are short; they'd make up much less than a quarter of a page of this book. Others are long; they'd make up about twelve hundred pages of this book. The chapters are grouped in volumes, called chromosomes. We have twenty-three pairs of chromosomes—a total of forty-six.

FROM GENES TO TRAITS TO HEALTH AND ILLNESS

When the body is ready to make proteins, it photocopies pages out of the instruction manual, that is, it transcribes the DNA. These copies are called RNA, short for ribonucleic acid. They're almost like the original, but not quite. The RNA gets sent out of the center of the cell—the nucleus where the DNA is stored—to the factories inside each cell that read the photocopied instruction manual and make protein. The protein then builds our cells, directs traffic, ushers and chaperones signaling molecules, helps with chemical reactions—basically creating the cell and then running the show.

So while genes code for our traits, like the color of our eyes, they also code for all the day-to-day things that make our cells work—for the transporters, messengers, enzymes, structural scaffolding, antibodies, and more. Within our bodies, they balance our fluids and nutrients, and make and maintain our body tissues such as muscle and bones and all the cells within our eyes. They are the building blocks of cells and tissue and, thus, of a living organism.

As we know, genes get passed on through heredity, but we have much more in common with each other than we may think. You and I share about 99.9 percent of the same genes. In fact, there is only about one-tenth (0.1) of a percent variability in genetic information from one person to the next. But while our instruction manuals are all pretty much the same, there are differences, as can be readily noticed in such ways as eye color, height, and ear shape.

More important, when it comes to health and illness, some of these chapters—these genes—have small errors—what we might call a typo in our book analogy—and as a result the proteins that they make don't work very well. Other times they have completely wrong instructions. Some of these genetic differences result in outright illness, such as sickle cell disease in which a single letter typo results in red blood cells that can't properly carry oxygen, are shaped like a sickle, and get stuck inside the blood vessels. This typo is often passed on from generation to generation.

Another example related to vision is retinitis pigmentosa, in which a child born with just one typo, or perhaps one of many different typos in several different chapters, results in creating protein—needed for proper retinal function—that doesn't work properly. Over years of constantly creating these defective proteins, the retina starts to malfunction, resulting in this retinal disorder. Sometimes this DNA typo gets passed along from generation to generation, but it can also appear on its own, as a new typo in a gene.

For protection against this (among other reasons), we all have two copies of each gene/chapter—one that we inherit from our mother and the other from our father. In many conditions, if a child inherits a typo from both the mother and father, then they'll have the same typo and the same illness. In other conditions, if a child inherits a typo from the mother but a normal set of instructions from the father, then the body can use the good instruction manual and create good protein—and no illness.

Sometimes even if you inherit one bad and one good set of instructions, the protein made by reading the chapter with the typo results in bad protein that contaminates everything, causing illness. It's like baking cake for a huge party of hundreds of people. You set aside the morning to make several batches of batter and the afternoon to bake them in the oven. You open up the chapter on batter mix, and you add a cup of flour, a cup of sugar, a stick of butter, two eggs, half cup of milk, a tad bit of baking powder, and some vanilla—and you mix it all together. You take a break and come back to make the next batch, and since we all have two copies of each chapter, this time you look at the other version of the cake mix recipe. Instead of saying a cup of s-u-g-a-r, it says a cup of s-a-l-t. You do exactly what it says. By the afternoon, you've made several batches, some from one chapter and some from the other. You combine them all together and start baking. Not surprisingly, your guests are not happy with their salty cake, and most of them go home ill.

Most of the time though, rather than malfunctioning or causing illness, typos in one of the chapters/genes result in proteins that are simply not quite as effective as they should be. And that's the essence of genetic susceptibility. Let's take macular degeneration. As we learned in chapter 2, this disease evolves from faulty instructions for proteins involved in inflammation or in sweeping up debris. Perhaps the typo translates into instructions for the flares that signal inflammatory cells, "Hey, here's where we need you." And if the flare is just a bit brighter than normal, you'll end up with more of the inflammatory warriors and a bit too much inflammation. Or the opposite may be true, and the typos code for a sweeper that is maybe ever so slightly slower, such that debris accumulates more easily. Over many decades, that may cause macular degeneration.

While some genetic traits don't automatically cause illness, they do make someone susceptible. Luckily, through good nutrition and healthy choices, you may be able to protect yourself from illness. A healthy balanced diet, for example, may help you control inflammation and decrease debris buildup in your retina—thus, decreasing the risk of macular degeneration. So while you can't change your genes, you can modify your nutrition and lifestyle and make other interventions to decrease your risk.

GENETIC TESTING

My friend—we'll call him Barry—is quite health-conscious. His mother has macular degeneration, and he, although still young, has some early signs of it. He read about how one-third of the population has a typo in a chapter that has instructions for one of the inflammatory genes for macular degeneration—complement factor H (CFH for short). He became even more worried when he read that if you had a typo in one of the two copies of the chapter for CFH, your risk for macular degeneration increased by two- to threefold and if you have a typo in both copies of the chapter for CFH, then your risk for macular degeneration increased by sevenfold!

Barry decided to take a genetic test that he understood was greater than 99 percent accurate—which indeed it was. He came to me with the results, which clearly stated "you're at risk," sure they were the game-losing clincher. I had to explain to him how genetic testing works.

Genetic testing looks for small typos. But at this point, commercially available testing doesn't search through all two billion words. It just picks chapters within a few volumes and looks for a few specific typos inside certain pages. It's like picking up this book, turning to a particular page, and making sure the word "cornea" is spelled correctly. But perhaps it's spelled "cornae"—well, we still know that was intended to be "cornea" and can probably continue with our reading. But if it was spelled "canoer"—same letters, but conveying a very different meaning, then maybe our body can't figure out what to do with the instructions, and the protein either comes out wrong or doesn't even come out at all.

I read the details of the testing very carefully. The science showed that it was indeed 99 percent accurate, and it was able to correctly find 92 percent of those tested who were indeed "at risk," thus missing only 8 percent of those "at risk." Furthermore, it correctly found 78 percent of those who are "not at risk" and identified them as such. But that number means that the test missed 22 percent of those who were *not* at risk and falsely identified them as being so. You may think perhaps that's ok—it's only 22 percent, and telling someone they're "at risk" when they're actually not may not be such a bad thing. Well is it?

Let's delve a little more into the statistics. Say we tested a thousand patients with early macular degeneration and we later found that fifty-five out of the one thousand patients progressed to severe macular degeneration (that's about the number we'd expect on average). At the time of testing, the genetic test finds 92 percent of those fifty-five patients who were "at risk" and then progressed to a severe form of the disease—that's fifty-one people. It only misses four—not bad! But out of the remaining 945 patients, the test correctly told 78 percent that they'd be fine but incorrectly identified 22 percent of them as "at risk" when they were not—that's 267 people. So out of the 318 positive test results (267 + 51), only fifty-one of them were truly positive; the other 267 were falsely positive. So while the test indeed is 99 percent accurate, a whopping 84 percent of the people who were scared with a "you're at risk" result were actually not at risk.

The message is that we're not yet at the point where we can offer good advice based on genetic testing. Over the past few years since Barry took the test, his eyes have been doing well, and he's had no progression. He trusts me, and we've put him on a good healthy nutrition plan that has made a difference in his overall health and well-being as well as his eyes. So just because a condition may run in your family or be a part of your genes, it doesn't mean you are doomed to suffer, even if you've already been diagnosed.

NUTRITION FOR MAKING AND REGULATING GENES

The primary focus of nutrition should be to ensure that your body—your cells, tissues, and organs—functions properly. Nutrition doesn't focus on fixing the bad genes or changing the typos, although science is getting close to repairing genes through a process called gene therapy. Genes have been fixed in beagles born with retinal gene defects, restoring vision where there was blinding retinal disease. It has shown promise in humans and may have a large role in improving vision in years to come. But there are some nutritional choices that can help out with your body's process of making and regulating its genetic information. For example, we know iron is essential in transporting oxygen throughout the body. But did you know it also helps in energy production and is essential for making DNA? A critical enzyme used in producing DNA for growing and dividing cells is dependent on iron to function properly. We're also learning more about how iron functions to help repair damage to DNA.

However, iron can cause oxidative damage, and if too much is taken it is so dangerous that it can be fatal, particularly to children. Its levels must be carefully balanced (see appendix for suggested dose ranges). Good natural sources for iron include nuts, steak, fish, eggs, tofu, beans of many types—navy, kidney, white, black-eyed, and lentils—beets, olives, carrots, and of course spinach.

Folate is a complexly structured nutrient that is also absolutely essential to making DNA. Back in 1931, while in Madras, India, British hematologist Dr. Lucy Wills first discovered a nutritional factor—later called folate—that both prevented and cured anemia, and since then we've learned a lot about how it works. Folate also helps maintain, prevent damage to, and repair our DNA by performing a unique chemical function of donating carbons in molecular reactions.

In addition, folate helps in the production of hemoglobin and acts as an indirect antioxidant by reducing the toxin homocysteine. When proteins are made—inside those protein-making factories located within our cells—they come out of the factories as what you can imagine to be thin strips of paper that need to be properly folded, just like origami. Proteins are made from protein-building blocks also known as amino acids. One amino acid, called homocysteine, is not used to make proteins, but rather acts like a bad joker, jumping in the wrong places and, as amino acid, jumping in to the protein-building process. Homocysteine causes the proteins to fold improperly, resulting in bad proteins that don't work too well. It also damages DNA and increases oxidative stress within cells.

Folate is widely recognized for its health benefits. It may decrease the risk of birth defects during pregnancy, prevent cancers, slow down the progression of Alzheimer's disease, and even reduce chronic fatigue. It can also help with eye disease. Remember the astronauts who developed eye conditions had lower levels of folate? Several research studies have shown a measurable decrease in the risk of cataracts associated with folate intake, and other studies have shown that it decreases the risk of retinal vein occlusions, stroke-like blood clots in the retina.

Oranges are well known for containing a lot of folate, but these foods contain even more folate in a 4-ounce serving: spinach, asparagus, collard greens, lettuce, broccoli, corn, kidney beans, black beans, lentils, and a wide variety of nuts such as walnuts, peanuts, pecans, and hazelnuts. Other good sources include okra, green beans, chickpeas, rice, and papaya.

NUTRITION FOR PREVENTING DNA DAMAGE

Folate is also required for the formation of another important nutrient called SAMe (pronounced like my friend Sammy, but with the accent on the second syllable). SAMe is short for s-adenosyl-methionine—what a mouthful! It helps prevent DNA damage and, research has suggested, it may also decrease the risk of certain types of cancer, as DNA damage can be a precursor to development of cancer. It also blocks inflammation; regulates enzymes; breaks down neural signaling molecules to balance their levels (and prevent overstimulation of neurons in a dangerous process called *excitotoxicity*, which may lead to glaucoma and other forms of neural injury); regulates the retina's response to light; forms the insulation—called myelin—that surrounds nerve fibers, including those that make up the optic nerve; and helps create our friend from chapter 1: alpha-lipoic acid, the antioxidant of antioxidants.

SAMe is unstable at room temperatures and is not a typical nutrient that you find in your diet. Your body can make its own SAMe, or you can supplement it with pills but be careful: A large portion of SAMe digested by mouth gets broken down into the toxin homocysteine in our livers. The best approach to increasing SAMe levels in your body is through a healthy balanced diet filled with folate-rich foods.

Vitamin B12—known as cobalamin—is also a very complexly structured nutrient. While it doesn't help in DNA production like folate or iron, it can protect DNA from damage through its essential involvement in pathways that lead to making DNA. By acting in these pathways, vitamin B12 also reduces the bad joker homocysteine and has been shown to protect neural cells from injury. It helps make energy and is required for maintenance of the nerve fiber myelin insulation.

Vitamin B12 is also essential for a cell's process of making a molecule called succinyl-CoA—you don't have to remember this molecule, but it is involved in building many other components of cells, such as the amino-acid protein–building blocks, the specialized phosphorus-containing lipids that make cell membranes, large ring-shaped molecules such as hemoglobin, and a whole host of neural signaling molecules, hormones, and steroids within our bodies. You can get your vitamin B12 from salmon, flounder, crabs, shrimp, steak, eggs, milk, yogurt, and cheese.

NUTRITION FOR ACTIVATING GENES

Gene activation is a name for the process of opening up the genetic instruction manual, turning to a specific chapter—the one on the gene of interest—and starting the process of making the protein from the instructions in that chapter. So if you want more brownies, then you'll need to turn to the chapter for the recipe. The body works the same way: If your body wants more of a certain protein, the gene needs to be "activated" (as in the related chapter in our book of genes must be read) to make that protein. This regulation of the DNA in our cells, which happens every millisecond as we speak, in turn leads to control of what proteins and how much of each are made inside our cells. It is very important to note that nutrients can control what genes are activated by cells in our body.

We previously learned about the importance and dangers of copper in oxidative damage. Copper also activates many genes to help keep the body healthy. Similarly, vitamin A has many roles we'll learn about as we continue—it also finds its way to the genetic cookbooks within our cells to activate genes, particularly those involved in the healthy growth of cells. By turning on specific genes, vitamin A can direct young, newly created cells to blossom into specific types of cells, whether that be immune defense cells or skin cells.

With good nutrition to turn on the right genes to promote eye health, you can begin protecting the genes that affect your vision, possibly preventing damage in the future. In the next section, we'll focus chapters on common and important vision-related conditions and diseases (macular degeneration, retinitis pigmentosa, diabetes, glaucoma, cataracts, and dry eye). I will explain the causes of each disorder and provide insight into how the eye functions both when it is well and when it is symptomatic of diseases. I'll also share details about what it's like to live with each condition, and which foods and nutrients have been shown, through clinical trials and medical research, to help alleviate symptoms and slow the progress of these conditions and diseases.

This part of the book is not just for those who have been diagnosed with or are predisposed to these disorders; anyone can benefit from learning how these disorders affect the eye, what preventative measures can be taken, and what insights researchers have learned about how we all can maintain our healthy vision.

SUMMARY 4: FEEDING YOUR GENES AND DNA THROUGHOUT YOUR LIFE

A gene consists of DNA that forms a code, like an instruction manual for how to build your cells, specifically how to make the proteins that run your cells.

Genes code for our traits and also code for all the day-to-day things that make our cells work: transporters, messengers, enzymes, structural scaffolding, antibodies, and more.

Genetic variations result in our traits—such as eye color or height—as well as illness and ailments.

Genetic variations can also result in genetic susceptibilities, which are caused by proteins that are not as effective as they should be.

So while you can't change your genes, your genes can be affected by your behavior: by what you eat, how active you are, and other lifestyle interventions.

Important nutrients from chapter 4:

- Iron—essential for making DNA and repairing damage to DNA.

- Folate—also essential for making and repairing DNA and decreases the toxin homocysteine.

- SAMe—prevents DNA damage.

- Vitamin B12—protects DNA from damage and reduces the toxin homocysteine.

- Copper—can activate (or turn on) specific genes to control which proteins and how much are made.

- Vitamin A—also activates genes, particularly involved in the healthy growth of cells.

PART II:

TREATING EYE CONDITIONS

CHAPTER 5
MACULAR DEGENERATION: WHEN THE CLEANERS STOP SWEEPING

When I go to a football game, I love watching the giant video screen—the Jumbotron, as some venues call it—because it reminds me of the eye. Both are composed of countless little parts, which all combine to create one image for us to see.

The Dallas Cowboys have the biggest Jumbotron in the United States, with some forty thousand LED bulbs making up a single, gigantic screen. Your eye has more than 125 million light-sensing cells, all working together to show you this page and the world around you. Let's pretend we're at the Cowboys' stadium, looking at the giant screen. If one or two of the forty thousand bulbs in that giant screen go out, we just won't notice it at all. But what if a group of five hundred bulbs in the center go out? Or one thousand? We'll probably notice a few blank spots in the image, which is about what happens when a condition called macular degeneration progresses.

But before we talk about macular degeneration, let's compare the Jumbotron to the layer of light-sensing cells of the eye—the retina. Instead of LED lights, your eye has what's called photoreceptors inside your retina (at the back of your eye). They form a layer of 125 million or so photoreceptors arranged like pixels on the flat screen of the Jumbotron. Their function is to receive light and share the image with your brain. If a scattered number of the photoreceptors start to die off, the brain is pretty good at covering up their minute blank spots—and is even pretty adept at covering up small groups of photoreceptors that are lost—but only up to a point.

Unfortunately, the catch is that when one photoreceptor dies off, it often affects its neighbors. These receive a signal that cells are dying, which in turn causes them to die, creating a brush-fire effect. Once a large group of photoreceptors is lost, the brain simply can't make up for that big blank spot. Even though we all have lots of photoreceptors (more than three thousand times the LED lights the Cowboys have), once the brush fire—called neurodegeneration in scientific terms—begins, it's very hard to stop. Eventually, the holes in one's vision get big enough to be noticeable, and once the patient comes to someone like me, the condition is diagnosed as macular degeneration.

However, unlike a Jumbotron where we can replace the LED lights when they burn out, we can't—yet—replace photoreceptors in the eye (even though some fish and reptiles can!). So ophthalmologists like me would prefer to catch and treat macular degeneration before it affects a patient's vision. We often do that, using nutrition to slow the progression of the disease.

WHAT CAUSES MACULAR DEGENERATION?

But before we discuss how to prevent macular degeneration, let's discuss how it's caused. Macular degeneration is a neurodegenerative disorder—a condition in which neurons degenerate or deteriorate—and photoreceptors are neurons. Neurodegeneration has become a buzzword in health care circles these days, largely because neurodegenerative diseases have been on the rise: Alzheimer's is one, Parkinson's (which actor Michael J. Fox has) is another, and ALS (Lou Gehrig's disease) is a third. All of these conditions take root in areas of our body that are very active, metabolically—Alzheimer's, Parkinson's, and ALS affect the brain; macular degeneration affects the retina.

The retina, as I've touched upon in previous chapters, is the most active part of your entire body and receives the most blood flow "per capita" of any organ, even more than your brain or heart. The macula—the center of the retina, the part that creates the center of your vision and the part affected by macular degeneration (hence the name)—is the most active component of the retina, and thus the absolute most active in the body, again even more so than your brain or heart.

Because it is so active, the macula produces a lot of "debris." This debris and waste includes the discs of the photoreceptors, which are shed each and every day. Photoreceptors contain up to a thousand discs arranged in layers to detect light particles called photons. As these discs are sloughed off each day, a layer of protecting cells—called the retinal pigment epithelium—cleans up: Each protecting cell packages and ingests around two thousand to four thousand discs daily from about thirty to forty adjacent photoreceptor cells. This task is colossal and complex for the cells and it can be easily overwhelmed by excess debris.

It's like having a restaurant that uses millions of dishes each day and each dishwasher (the protecting cell in our analogy) has thousands of dishes to wash. If washers break down or if there are excess dirty dishes, then the dirty dishes start to pile up. Likewise, as you get older, your eye starts to slow down and simply can't clean up the mess quickly enough—so the debris produced stays there, or even increases in its production (thus accelerating the problem), or both. We call that debris *drusen*, after the Greek word for bump, because that's what it looks like under the microscope.

Drusen: Debris Behind the Retina

When scientists first discovered drusen around 1850, they didn't quite know what they were. But today, we understand the origins of drusen and how they can harm the eyes. When you look at drusen under a microscope, they often look like pale bumps underneath the retina. If you picture a large translucent tarp on the ground, covering up pale yellow upside-down dinner plates in the center, that's pretty close to what I see when I look at a patient who has them, given, of course, that the scale is far smaller and drusen vary vastly in shape.

I spent some years of my career simply looking at drusen through a machine called an OCT (optical coherence tomography). The OCT is pretty cool, as far as ophthalmology machines go: It bounces light off the retina and creates images similar to what you see in an ultrasound. But because the OCT uses light energy rather than sound energy (what an ultrasound uses), I can see five microns of resolution—which is a really sharp picture of this truly tiny part of the body (by comparison a human hair is about one hundred microns in thickness on average). I recently wrote a medical book geared toward other eye doctors, called *Atlas of OCT: Retinal Anatomy in Health and Pathology,* in which I describe eight different kinds of drusen, which live in three broad locations behind the retina, using this new imaging technique. But what you should know about drusen is that there are many variations, which is important when it comes to your doctor detecting drusen and predicting what types of damage they may cause.

The sheer presence of drusen causes a lot of problems for the retina, which in turn may affect vision. First and foremost, the drusen often contain a residue called lipofuscin, which in the presence of light and oxygen results in the production of toxic oxidants (the effects of which you learned about in chapter 1). Of course light exposure is high in the retina, and the highest amount of oxygen consumption of any tissue in the body occurs in the retina— remember, this is the most active part of your body—so the retina is particularly susceptible to oxidative damage from the drusen. In addition, the drusen may cause inflammation (the effects of which you learned about in chapter 2). But more specific to the retina, scientists including myself have found that the accumulation and presence of drusen may deprive the retina of the oxygen, nutrients, and blood flow that it needs to stay healthy.

Even worse, because drusen contain broken-down proteins and fats and even minerals and elements, they may limit the retina's ability to control and dispose of its waste. The end result is that the cells of the retina start to degenerate, or malfunction, and eventually die off, turning off the LED lights of our retina one by one, starting that neurodegeneration brush fire.

As macular degeneration progresses, small blind spots can grow to larger patches, and blurred vision can develop. Distortions in vision come from having drusen—a bump or many irregular bumps—behind the Jumbotron distorting the picture. In severe cases of macular degeneration, loss of vision and blindness can occur. Though we've known about macular degeneration since the nineteenth century, more recent research has taught us more. One of the largest and most important studies about macular degeneration was conducted in the all-American, small midwestern town of Beaver Dam, Wisconsin, starting in the late 1980s. Since that time, the National Institutes of Health (NIH) has sponsored nearly three hundred studies on eye disease in and around Beaver Dam, including one that studied macular degeneration and drusen specifically. Of the five thousand people between the ages of forty-three and eighty-four who participated, over 95 percent had drusen in at least one of their eyes—that's nearly everyone! Even more important, the study found that more than one-third of participants over age seventy-five showed the kind of changes and drusen accumulation that qualifies as macular degeneration, and nearly one in ten of the participants under age fifty-five did.

There are about eight million people with severe or moderate macular degeneration and likely millions more who either go undiagnosed and/or live with mild symptoms. Even though most patients with macular degeneration do not go blind, by all accounts, macular degeneration is a leading cause of blindness in the United States.

DRY AND WET MACULAR DEGENERATION

There are two different kinds of macular degeneration: dry and wet. Ninety percent of people with macular degeneration have the dry kind, which is what we'll mostly discuss in this chapter. The 10 percent of people who have wet macular degeneration essentially have the dry kind plus cracks in their retina through which abnormal blood vessels grow. It's like having weeds grow through cracks in your sidewalk, except that these weeds bleed, leak fluid, and scar the retina, causing irreparable damage to the photoreceptors in the retina and often rapid vision loss.

WHO'S AT RISK

So, who is at risk for macular degeneration? And how can we treat, or even prevent, it?

The truth is, we don't entirely know yet. One theory in today's scientific community is that macular degeneration isn't just one disease but perhaps one of hundreds, even thousands, of distinct eye conditions we group together. As someone who has been studying macular degeneration in its many forms and iterations for years, I believe in this theory. However, there are certainly defined risk factors, proven treatments, and healthy preventative measures that can help people make informed choices.

Let's begin by sharing what I know about the risk factors for macular degeneration. The biggest one is age—as you get older, your cells do too. So that's why it's often called age-related macular degeneration. Most macular degeneration is age-related. As we detailed in chapter 1, the degeneration of your entire body is more likely when you are eighty-five than when you are forty-five or even seventy-five. Unfortunately, we can't turn back time.

But what about genetics—your genes? There is an association between ethnicity and macular degeneration: in Caucasians, for example, the risk of having the severe form of macular degeneration is four times higher than the general population of Americans, and in Native Americans, the risk is sixteen times higher. Genetic differences are believed to be the reason for the higher risk among certain ethnic groups. Our genes define the color of our eyes (our iris color) and several studies have suggested that people with lighter iris or eye color (particularly those with blue eyes) could have a higher risk of macular degeneration—but the jury is still out. What we do know is that a family history of this condition may indicate a gene that *predisposes* you to the risk—it does not necessarily mean that you will develop the condition, but you are much more likely to encounter it than everyone else. Nutrition may help decrease that risk.

There are many other risk factors, such as smoking (which nearly doubles your risk) and obesity, primarily due to the risk factors of obesity itself: high blood pressure, high cholesterol, heart disease, and poor nutrition, all of which increase your risk of macular degeneration.

And what about sunlight? One study examined eight hundred watermen who worked for years on the Chesapeake Bay catching Maryland crabs and fish. I live near the Chesapeake myself and know that while the sun shining down on the water is gorgeous, if you take your sunglasses off for even a second, you'll find yourself squinting because of all the light hitting your eyes at once from the sunlight above and the reflected sunlight from the water. Despite being out in this blinding sun day after day, the study found that the fisherman had no damage to their retinas from the UV light. Instead, they shared an increased risk for macular degeneration from excess high-energy *blue* light. So what is this light and how do we avoid it?

HOW LIGHT CAN DAMAGE THE RETINA

When we hear about sunlight, most of us worry about ultraviolet or UV light. However, the eye does a wonderful job protecting the retina from UV light, which comes in three forms: UV-A, UV-B, and UV-C. (These three kinds of damaging UV light are distinguished by their wavelengths.) Lucky for us, though, your cornea blocks 100 percent of all UV-C light, 40 percent of UV-B, and 20 percent of UV-A light. The natural lens in your eyes blocks 99 percent of UV-B and 99 percent of UV-A light, leaving an extremely small amount of UV light that hits your retinas.

What does reach the retina and is damaging to it is what's called high-energy blue light. This light is visible (we can see it) and, as the name suggests, has a blue color. The vast amount of high-energy blue light in sunlight causes photo-oxidation, a fancy word that basically means this light is feeding the oxidation process that ages your retina, as described in chapter 1. So even though your eyes are protecting your retinas from UV light, the high-energy blue light gets through. That's what the watermen study showed: Excess outdoor sunlight exposure can perhaps double the risk for macular degeneration. While what defines as "excessive" is up for discussion, wearing sunglasses—especially those that have dark or amber filters to decrease the blue light—certainly could help.

Natural Sunglasses

In addition to wearing sunglasses when outdoors—or a brimmed hat, or both—perhaps the most controllable risk factor for macular degeneration (and overall eye health) is your diet. Research has overwhelmingly shown how certain nutrients, particularly lutein and zeaxanthin, can protect your retina from damage that eventually creates drusen and causes macular degeneration.

Lutein and zeaxanthin actually give eyes their own natural sunglasses. As most of us know, sunlight can burn—just ask anyone who has sat on a beach without sunscreen. Worse yet, our eye acts like a magnifying glass, with the lens of the eye focusing light on the retina. It reminds me of when I was a child, holding up a magnifying glass to the sun and burning a hole in a leaf. Our retinas can easily heat up past the core temperature of 98.6° to 104°. So how does the eye protect itself? It does so by using blood flow to cool the retina to a relatively chilly 98.6° and with nutrients like lutein and zeaxanthin, which absorb the high-energy blue light that hurt the watermen's eyes and yours. Our retinas have their own layer of lutein and zeaxanthin in front that act as "natural sunglasses" and absorb roughly 40 to 90 percent of all the high-energy blue light you see—before it even hits the photoreceptors in your retina, thus helping to keep it cool (and burn free). The retina has the highest concentration of these nutrients in our bodies, and their light-filtering effects even improve image quality.

It's a pretty amazing process, but unfortunately not everyone eats enough lutein or zeaxanthin to have blue light protection every time you step out into the sun. But you should, especially if you carry any of the risk factors for macular degeneration.

The nutrients that give us "natural sunglasses," lutein and zeaxanthin, are carotenoids, organic pigments that only occur naturally in plants. Other carotenoids—out of hundreds known and others unknown—while not "natural sunglasses" are powerful antioxidants: lycopene (found in tomatoes) and beta-carotene (found in carrots). You can find lutein and zeaxanthin in leafy greens like kale, spinach, and romaine lettuce. Other sources include brussels sprouts, squash, tomatoes, raspberries, peas, and broccoli; see appendix for more.

In addition to their antioxidant and light-absorbing capabilities, carotenoids can help slow the development of cancer by stabilizing certain proteins that, if destroyed, begin creating cancer cells. Carotenoids may also help lower cholesterol, by interfering in the pathway within the body that they share (causing a cholesterol traffic jam of sorts) or by inhibiting cholesterol-forming enzymes. Also, carotenoids are believed to prevent the oxidation of fats in blood vessels, a process that would lead to atherosclerosis, blood vessel cholesterol clots and plaques that can result in heart disease and stroke, as well as artery or vein clots in the retina or optic nerve strokes. *And* carotenoids play an essential role in immune protection. So it's not just macular degeneration that carotenoids are good for.

If you are at risk, try to include plants that have carotenoids—particularly those containing lots of lutein and zeaxanthin—in your diet at least daily. As we'll learn in chapter 7, you'll need to balance these nutrients with others to help the molecules—the "good" HDL cholesterol—that transport the lutein and zeaxanthin to the retina. But like all eye diseases (and really, health in general), there isn't a one-size-fits-all solution. What I can offer is this: Scientific evidence has shown that eating several nutrients on a regular basis, *especially in combination with one another*, can decrease existing risk factors and potentially even slow the progression of the disease once it's started.

DRUSEN DESTROYERS

The 5 "drusen destroyers" that keep retinas healthy are phytic acid, carnitine, coenzyme Q10, chromium, and methionine.

1. **Phytic acid**—also known as phytate, inositol hexaphosphate, or IP6—binds metals that can create oxidative damage. It is a

precursor to IP3, also known as inositol triphosphate, which signals the cells behind the retina to clean up debris. The best sources are beans—particularly soybean tofu, lentils, navy beans, white beans, and chickpeas—and grains such as wild rice, whole wheat bread, and whole wheat pasta—as well as some vegetables such as spinach and carrots, and nuts.

2. **Carnitine** is a compound formed from amino acids (the building blocks of proteins); 95 percent of your body's supply of carnitine is found in the muscles and heart, although it does live in the lens of the eye. Carnitine has been shown to help remove debris in the retina, the main cause of macular degeneration, and even reverse the progress of the disease (though so far the research has been limited to a single study in Italy). The best sources for carnitine are steak, ground beef, milk, ice cream, and cod.

3. **Coenzyme Q10** (known as "vitamin Q") is an antioxidant that helps preserve vitamin E in cell membranes. It is a very important nutrient that helps cells produce energy, and it is especially beneficial in retina-related diseases such as macular degeneration because it helps specific organelles—called lysosomes—inside cells produce acid so that they can digest debris. Like carnitine, coenzyme Q10 is primarily found in meat, including ground beef and chicken, but also in fish such as sardines, mackerel, and yellowtail, and nuts such as pistachios.

4. **Chromium:** In chapter 7 on diabetes, we'll talk more about chromium, but little is known about how this essential metallic element works in the body—it is believed to interact with

cell signaling messengers. We do know that it works with the amino acid methionine to help remove debris from behind the retina. The two top sources for chromium are fish, particularly haddock, and broccoli. Other meats, vegetables, and fruits contain smaller amounts.

5. **Methionine:** This amino acid helps boost energy inside cells and is a precursor to antioxidants such as glutathione and SAMe (which we learned about in chapters 1 and 4 respectively). With the help of chromium, it can help remove debris from behind the retina. Methionine can be found in meats, dairy products, nuts, and soybeans (careful, though, as methionine can easily turn into that toxic joker homocysteine).

Clinical studies have shown all these nutrients help keep retinas healthy—a proven preventative measure for macular degeneration—and can also help avoid and treat other diseases of the retina, eye, or even throughout the body in general. The more the medical community learns about nutrients, the more we realize that most are good for your entire body, in addition to helping one particular part (in this case, the retina).

A PARTICULARLY HEALTHY DIET

Recently, the world's oldest-ever human in documented history— born in 1897—died at the age of 116. He was Japanese—and he reportedly ate pumpkins and sweet potatoes three times each day. These foods are tremendously high in carotenoids and other nutrients. Some of the longest living people are from Okinawa, Japan, and their diets are low in meats, except for fish, and high in vegetables, particularly sweet potatoes. In addition to Okinawa, the island of Sardinia in Italy and Costa Rica in Central America have been called "Blue Zones"—a term that came up when mapping longevity in Sardinia, indicating areas of locals with long life spans and carotenoid-rich diets.

The lesson is a healthy diet of wholesome foods is essential for your health and well-being. We have included easy-to-reference charts at the end of this book with specific foods and why they are helpful. But I think the best way to make sure you are eating the right nutrients is to take a balanced approach and eat as many different fruits and vegetables as you can. By incorporating a wide variety of produce in your diet, your body will receive different kinds of nutrients.

In addition to the drusen destroyers, there are also vitamins and minerals that people suffering from or at risk for macular degeneration should try to include in their diet. Macular degeneration involves aging and oxidative damage, so we need to eat the antioxidants mentioned in chapter 1. Research has also shown that inflammation, either from the drusen discussed earlier or from other sources, causes macular degeneration to worsen, so to fight macular degeneration you should eat the nutrients mentioned in chapter 2 on inflammation. Prevention of macular degeneration requires maintaining good blood flow (as discussed in chapter 3) and regulation of protective genes (as discussed in chapter 4). Vitamin A, vitamin C, vitamin E, and zinc should also be in your list of vitamins to make sure are in your diet. But, as I've said before, it is always smarter and safer to eat your nutrients through wholesome foods instead of popping pills—and it will be harder to overdose on any one nutrient, vitamin, or mineral.

OVERDOSE DANGER:
VITAMINS AND OTHER NUTRIENTS

"Can I overdose on vitamins?" is a question I'm often asked by patients. Yes it's possible, even probable for some people taking nutrients in pills—however, taking too much of a good thing in the form of wholesome foods is relatively harmless *most of the time.*

A great example of too-much-of-a-good-thing is vitamin E. Though it's a powerful antioxidant that, at the proper dose, can protect the retina and may protect against macular degeneration, high doses can cause diarrhea, bloating, fatigue—and also block antioxidants that are equally as beneficial for preventing macular degeneration. Too much vitamin E can hinder your body's ability to absorb vitamins A, D, and K, thus resulting in lower levels of them in your system. More important, taking too much vitamin E can increase the risk of bleeding in the eye and increase the risk for stroke. So while you should eat vitamin-E-rich foods such as almonds, sunflower seeds and hazelnuts, be wary of any supplement that has you absorbing more than 100–150 milligrams (mg) per day.

One patient whom I'll call Sharon has an eye condition called cone-rod dystrophy. While not macular degeneration, it is a retinal degeneration where photoreceptors are slowly lost—it blurs her central vision and she has trouble seeing at night. An orthodox Jew, she came to see me when she began having trouble reading from her evening prayer book. In addition, she has experienced dry eye.

Sharon takes a broad-spectrum multivitamin that contains a moderate amount of vitamin E (100 IU) and contains vitamin A (3500 IU). Recently, her internist put her on 800 IU of vitamin E, to keep her skin healthy. Vitamin E at this dose blocks the absorption of vitamin A from the gut and also interferes with the conversion of vitamin A in the retina into the light-sensing pigments of the retina. The result? Less light-sensing pigment and abnormal accumulation of vitamin A in the cells behind the retina, causing damage to the photoreceptors. The vitamin E excess caused by her skin supplement thus resulted in decreased retina function, and in a vitamin A deficiency that caused dry eye! Her main eye doctor, who is my friend and a rabbi, called me as soon as he found out what was going on, and we took her off the extra vitamin E but kept her on the broad-spectrum multivitamin, which she supplemented with a healthy diet, including fruits and vegetables. Her ability to read at night has improved to how it was before she started the supplemental vitamin E.

Zinc

Another great example of a nutrient that can, at high levels, be hazardous is zinc. The second most abundant trace metal in the human body, the highest concentration of zinc is in the eye, especially in the retina and macula. Zinc is necessary for the action of over one hundred enzymes, particularly those needed for essential function of the retina, such as sensing light, sending signals between neurons, and removing debris. Zinc, along with its metal buddy copper, protects the retina from light damage by helping form and binding to a pigmented chemical substance called melanin. Because zinc is important for the health of the macula, supplements of zinc in the diet may slow the process of macular degeneration.

However, zinc in high doses acts as an oxidant. As a study I published recently in the *Journal of Neuroscience* shows, early zinc accumulation is the first step in apoptosis, or cell death, in neurons, which in turn is a precursor of vision loss in macular degeneration. Although some studies show a moderate level of zinc can prevent and even slow the progression of macular degeneration among some patients, different studies prove it causes oxidation and disease if patients have high levels of zinc in their diet. Your best course of action is to incorporate zinc into your diet through zinc-rich foods such as nuts, dairy, and beans.

Eye Vitamins

Perhaps you've heard the advertisements for the over-the-counter "eye vitamins"—pills that target your eye health. Many of these pills contain high amounts of zinc and vitamin E, and they cite data from the famous AREDS medical study (Age-Related Eye Disease Study). These data showed that taking a pill (that contained 500 mg vitamin C, 400 IU vitamin E, 15 mg beta-carotene, 80 mg zinc, and 2 mg copper) lowered the risk of severe worsening of macular degeneration by about 25 percent, but only in people who already had "higher-risk" macular degeneration. It is a wonderfully important study that provided a strong rationale for the use of nutrients in macular degeneration. However, the pills did not appear to benefit anyone with milder or no macular degeneration. Also, with such high doses of vitamin E and zinc, are the potential benefits of these so-called "eye vitamins" worth taking the risk of overloading on vitamin E and zinc? It's important to remember that nutrient pills should be considered medicines. As we learned earlier, high amounts of vitamin E and zinc can be damaging. Advertisements promoting eye vitamins based on the AREDS data don't mention the related risks. Buried in the AREDS data itself is a single sentence identifying a threefold increased risk of circulatory system side effects (changes in blood pressure or even stroke) from the zinc.

Moreover, looking at the study's observation of a decreased risk of severe worsening of macular degeneration that occurred in *some* patients, how did they determine when the macular degeneration got worse? By taking photographs of the retina, *not* by a doctor examining the patient. Would you ever want someone diagnosing you as having macular degeneration without any doctor ever having examined you? In addition, the photographs date to the mid- to late-1990s—today, image quality and our ability to detect macular degeneration are both more advanced. So perhaps we should be cautious in interpreting the results. Perhaps we should think twice before taking an "eye vitamin" with such high risks and perhaps none of the benefits you really expect.

You may hear that the latest AREDS data—called AREDS 2—fixed the problems with the previous study by evaluating reduced zinc, for example. However, we didn't glean as much information from the study as we had wanted, as the study was divided into sixteen groups, a very large quantity that would require a tremendous number of patients to really parse out what works and what doesn't. The study essentially found that *adding* lutein and zeaxanthin or adding omega-3 oils (we'll learn more about those in chapter 6) to the original formula provided no additional benefit—but that doesn't mean that no benefit actually exists. It did suggest that taking lutein and zeaxanthin in pills was better than not taking them—although only if you were unable to enjoy a good diet full of fruits and vegetables high in lutein and zeaxanthin.

As always, a balanced approach is a healthy approach. What we are finding out, as shown by a 2014 study on macular degeneration, is that a healthy diet full of fruits, vegetables, grains, nuts, fish, and steamed or boiled chicken is associated with lower rates of advanced macular degeneration. So as I've said before and will say again, it's always better to *eat* vitamins and minerals than to swallow them in pill form—you'll get a broader spectrum of nutrients and better levels. However, if you have any questions or doubts about what nutrients you're getting from your diet, talking with your doctor about supplementing with specific pills if needed can be a smart move.

Healthful foods most often will go a long way to helping your whole body, not just your eyes. If you're looking to combat macular degeneration, do so with the vitamins that are proven to help, and eat a wide variety of nutritious foods. And keep in mind that the same nutrients that help protect our eyes against macular degeneration can help in a wide variety of eye conditions, including other retinal ailments, such as retinitis pigmentosa, which we'll learn about next. And nutrients that help in retinitis pigmentosa and other eye conditions can help in macular degeneration.

SUMMARY 5: MACULAR DEGENERATION

Macular degeneration is a neurodegenerative disorder of the light-sensing retina.

Debris called drusen accumulates behind the retina in macular degeneration.

Drusen cause oxidative damage, inflammation, deprive the retina of oxygen and nutrients, and limit the retina's ability to dispose of its waste.

Risk factors for macular degeneration: age, ethnicity, smoking, obesity, high blood pressure, high cholesterol, heart disease, excess high-energy blue light in sunlight, and poor nutrition.

Important nutrients from chapter 5:

- Lutein and zeaxanthin—plant pigments that protect the retina from sunlight damage.
- Phytic acid—binds metal and signals cells behind the retina to clean up debris.
- Carnitine—an amino acid that helps remove debris in the retina.
- Coenzyme Q10—a nutrient that helps cells produce energy.
- Chromium—a metal that interacts with cell signaling messengers.
- Methionine—an amino acid that is a precursor to antioxidants.

- Zinc—supports the retina in sensing light, sending signals, removing debris, and forming the pigment melanin.

The top debris-reducing nutrients are: phytic acid, carnitine, coenzyme Q10, chromium, and methionine.

Excess vitamin E can block absorption of vitamins A, D, and K, interfere with conversion of vitamin A to the retina's light-sensing pigments, and increase the risk of bleeding.

Excess zinc is toxic and can cause oxidation.

CHAPTER 6
RETINITIS PIGMENTOSA: A GENE THAT STEALS SIGHT

You may remember the very pious monk Father Gregor Mendel, from the mid 1800s, as the founder of modern genetics. He cultivated more than twenty-nine thousand pea plants and identified some basic principles of inheritance. After the peas, he studied honeybees, and created a strain—bred from a combination of South American and Egyptian honeybees—that produced a reportedly delectable blend of honey. What he and many others soon found was that these honeybees were so ferocious that they started attacking many monks in the monastery and even stung villagers many miles away. They had to destroy those hives.

As we learned in chapter 4, a gene is the unit of heredity in any living organism. We've learned a lot about genetics since 1869, when Swiss physician Friedrich Miescher isolated DNA from the pus stuck on discarded bandages. In 1953 James Watson and Francis Crick discovered the structure of DNA and later received a Nobel Prize for their revolutionary work. In 1990 the Human Genome Project began, and it took a short thirteen years, until 2003, to identify—to "sequence"—the three billion DNA subunits in the whole human genome and discover the twenty- to twenty-five thousand human genes. So now that we've discovered all the genes, do we think the rest is history? Not at all. Each population holds a stunning diversity of variation in appearance, behavior and—importantly—in susceptibility to disease. What makes this tremendous variation is the genetic basis of the human.

GENETICS AND RETINITIS PIGMENTOSA

Despite the intense genetics research over the last two decades, we still have our work cut out for us. Take for example, a disorder of the retina, the light-sensing part of the eye. The disease is called retinitis pigmentosa (or RP). Unlike the other conditions in this book, RP begins in childhood. The onset of this disease gives patients a similar sensation to what most of us feel when walking into a dark movie theater on a sunny day—but for patients with RP, the adjustment takes much more time to make. Because RP patients are sensitive to changes in light, moving around during twilight can be very hard for them. As the condition advances, peripheral vision (the ability of a patient to see on the side) diminishes, creating a sort of tunnel vision that in later stages becomes complete blindness.

RP is usually diagnosed when a patient comes to the office complaining of these symptoms—as we look in the back of the eye at the retina, we see the telltale signs. A specialized test, called the electroretinogram (like an EKG of the heart) looks at the electric signals generated by the retina—since the light-sensing cells of the retina convert light to chemical and then electrical signals. With RP it shows decreased function of the rods and often cones in the retina.

RP is a neurodegeneration of the retina, just like macular degeneration, that starts in childhood instead of adulthood—affecting about one hundred thousand people here in the United States. It is dictated by genetic defects resulting in loss of the light-sensing cells of the retina: the rods and cones. It causes a slow, progressive loss of rods and then cones.

From laboratory research over many years, we have come to understand quite a lot about the genetics of RP: Defects in nearly two hundred genes that manifest the same clinical disease have been identified and numerous animal models with RP exist and have been studied extensively. However, despite all the knowledge of the

71

genetics of RP, and all the scientific studies on RP and developing treatments, at the moment there are no cures and there are no effective medical interventions or medicines, other than nutrition to slow its progress. We really understand little—from a molecular and cellular basis—about how the condition actually progresses.

Just as macular degeneration is probably not one condition but a group of many similar diseases, RP is probably a group of similar diseases that result in the clinical condition we call RP. A few years ago, I coined the term "retinal ciliopathy" to group together a set of similar conditions in which numerous different types of gene defects cause a cell organelle—called the cilium—to improperly function. This cilium is found in various places in the body, including the rods and cones of the retina, to connect the light-sensing part of these photoreceptors to the signaling part. Defects in the gene that codes for the cilium results in an abnormal cilium in the photoreceptors, causing them to malfunction and die off over time. This results in one of the forms of RP—defects in other types of cell structures and proteins cause other forms of RP.

Defective proteins simply do not function properly—whether in the membrane of the cell, the nucleus of the cell, or in the organelles of the cell—or they just block the traffic and flow of other proteins in the cells. The result is that the cell malfunctions and starts to degenerate and die off. Photoreceptors in humans, unlike skin cells, do not regrow when they have been lost, although photoreceptors constantly regenerate themselves in some fish and some amphibians! We hope that one day we can unlock in our eyes the same stem cells that exist in these fish and amphibians—and they do indeed exist inside our own eyes—and direct them to grow into new photoreceptors to replenish ones that degenerate. Until then, what can we do for RP? So far, nutrition works the best.

RP is a devastating disease for those who suffer from it. One of my young patients—an avid basketball player we'll call Valerie—was bumping into things at night and her peripheral vision was also decreased. Her parents brought her in to see me, and we determined she had RP. I've been seeing her for several years, and after changing her diet to include specific nutritional components, her function at night and her side vision improved a bit, despite our expectation that they would worsen over time. Her results are not typical—it's more common for changes in diet to slow down the progression.

INEFFECTIVE TREATMENT OPTIONS FOR RP

As with many devastating diagnoses, those with RP will often try anything, however unsuccessful. In a quaint town outside of London, just a few decades ago, people with RP were lining up to enter a cage full of specially bred bees. The nape of their neck would remain exposed so that the bee stings could be concentrated in that area. Well-educated and well-intentioned folk would respond that their vision improved, but the reality is that the treatment did not work.

Not too long ago in Russia, amniotic membrane from placentas was used as a treatment for RP, as was genetic material extracted from yeast. Even more recently, in Cuba, ozone therapy often with electrostimulation has been promoted. Yes, electrostimulation, as in shock with electricity, followed by pumping toxic ozone gas into the bloodstream. All this talk of snake oil is worrisome; those who are afflicted by these blinding conditions often find themselves desperate for a solution.

FISH OIL: A VIABLE TREATMENT OPTION

The Japanese have probably come closest to a remedy: fish—and specifically fish oil. Old age and Japanese are often synonymous.

The Japanese eat a healthy, low-fat diet, but the fat they do consume comes from fish oils. Perhaps you remember those smelly fish oil pills—or perhaps you take some now, although these days, they're formulated and packaged to be not as smelly as before.

Why are fish oils important? Well, all human brain cells, nerve cells, and retinal cells are made of more than 70 percent fat, much of it a special kind of fat called fatty acids. Fatty acids are found in all sorts of oils, from canola to corn oil, from sunflower to safflower oil, from animal fat to fish oils. Common fats are a combination of fatty acids joined with a sugar-alcohol backbone to form a triglyceride—which you may have heard of, as some are saturated fats and some are unsaturated fats. So there are two types of essential fatty acids: omega-3 and omega-6 fatty acids—originally called vitamin F until they were discovered to be fats. Sometimes they're simply called omega-3 and -6 oils. There is also a third type: omega-9 oils. All three differ in molecular configuration, which gives them very different properties. They also differ because the body can make the omega-9 oils it needs—so it is not called an "essential" fatty acid, versus omega-3 and -6 oils, which are called "essential" fatty acids because these need to come from our diets.

Omega-3 oils are typically referred to as the good fatty acids while omega-6 oils are the "bad" ones, found in chocolate chip cookies as well as cheese, meats, and crackers. These omega-6 oils promote inflammation, blood clotting, and abnormal blood vessel growth. But as we will learn in chapter 10, omega-6 oils are actually good for you, when balanced with omega-3 oils. As we know by the name—essential fatty acids—omega-6 oils are essential to our good health.

Let's get back to the omega-3 oils. These fatty acids form the cell membranes, they anchor proteins in these membranes, they send signals within cells, and they turn on and off specific genes, particularly those involved in the metabolism and healthy growth of cells.

Omega-3 oils are involved in many processes throughout the body and are believed to decrease heart disease, improve blood flow, reduce cholesterol, help prevent stroke, decrease inflammation, and block growth of abnormal blood vessels. And omega-3 oils are essential for the retina. The light-sensing portion of photoreceptors is arranged in discs that look like stacks of pancakes, hundreds of pancakes high—up to a thousand—with light-sensing particles embedded within the surface of each pancake—think blueberries on the surface of each pancake in the stack of the hundreds of pancakes. Now, in the eye, these discs—pancakes—are transparent. A single particle of light—called a photon—comes down from above and goes right through the pancakes until it hits a blueberry and triggers that blueberry to send a message down to the frying pan the pancakes are sitting in. In the actual cell, the signal gets transferred to the body of the photoreceptor cell, which then sends the signal to other neurons of the retina through synapses using neurotransmitters. If these pancakes are liquidy—not fully cooked—then the blueberries can float around. When the pancake gets cooked, the blueberries get fixed in place. In the photoreceptor discs, the omega-3 oils make the membranes of these discs "fluidic"—liquidy—so that the light-sensing pigments and other components of the membranes can move around, enabling them to respond faster to light stimuli and get replaced faster once they are used up. That's why much more than half and up to 90 percent of the membrane of these photoreceptor discs is fatty acids.

One of the most important of these special oils, called docosahexaenoic acid—DHA for short—is found in fish oils. DHA is a fatty acid that is highest in brain tissue—in fact the highest concentration of DHA anywhere in our body is in the photoreceptor cells of the retina.

Numerous research studies have demonstrated the benefits of omega-3 oils and DHA, which are very important in the development of the eye in infants (and the developing brain). That is why breast milk and certain brands of infant formula contain high amounts of DHA. They may decrease the risk and severity of dry eye. A few studies have shown that they may decrease the risk of macular degeneration, and one study found in people with macular degeneration, the drusen can actually decrease in those who took a concoction consisting of omega-3 oils, the drusen buster carnitine, and coenzyme Q10—and their vision improved! This kind of reversal of macular degeneration is extraordinary— what we all hope for. And there's good reason to believe that it may be replicated in future studies.

In RP, more than a handful of clinical trials have looked at the effects of omega-3 oils and DHA, and while the jury is still out, there is evidence to demonstrate a slowing of the progression of RP in those who take omega-3 oils and DHA. As such, many eye doctors will recommend these fatty acids for patients with RP. Just a caution: Very high amounts of omega-3 oils increase the risk of bleeding by blocking platelet activities. Diabetics should use caution as omega-3 oils can increase blood sugars. Milder side effects of omega-3 oils include upset stomach, heartburn, abdominal bloating, diarrhea, and skin rashes.

Sources for Omega-3 Oils and DHA

Top sources for DHA include freshwater fish such as trout and cold-water ocean fish such as salmon. However, be careful as some of the larger ocean fish—such as mackerel, tuna, shark, and swordfish— often contain high amounts of mercury, a toxic metal. The FDA and EPA have guides about what fish to avoid; you can also ask your fishmonger or seafood provider at the grocery store.

Other sources for omega-3 oils include rockfish, sardines, and anchovy, as well as walnuts, flaxseed, cheeses, tofu, turkey, and grains.

CAROTENOIDS AND VITAMIN A

Some seafood contains more benefits than just from the omega-3 oils. Krill oil, for example, is a wonderful source of omega-3 oils as well as a powerful antioxidant called astaxanthin. It's a carotenoid that is not restricted to production in plants but instead is made by some marine species: krill, shrimp, salmon, trout, and algae. It's what gives these sea creatures (and red algae) their red color. Krill and arctic shrimp are among the very best sources of astaxanthin—orders of magnitude better than salmon or trout.

While there are hundreds of different types of carotenoids, in general, carotenoids are derived from plants. They are pigments in the plants, like the powerful antioxidant lycopene, the red carotenoid found in tomatoes, watermelon, and grapefruit. Often overlooked are crocin and crocetin, which come from saffron, that little yellow spice that is the most expensive spice in the world. Saffron is also loaded with other carotenoids and is a powerful antioxidant, and there is good reason to believe that it can protect retinal cells from injury.

Beta-carotene is the orange carotenoid found in carrots, pumpkin, sweet potatoes, cantaloupe, and apricots. Some greens—such as collards, kale, and spinach—are also high in beta-carotene despite hiding the orange color. Although beta-carotene is converted to vitamin A in the body, don't worry about eating too many carrots, because a good healthy liver can limit this conversion. For most, too many carrots will simply cause your skin to turn orangey in color—but be careful if you are a smoker. One study (which incidentally was a cancer prevention study) showed that too much vitamin A and/or beta-carotene can increase the risk of developing lung cancer.

Because vitamin A is required for the pigment to be produced in the retinal photoreceptors, it is needed for our retinas to function well. Some thirty-four hundred years ago ancient Egyptians used liver, which is full of vitamin A, to treat night-blindness, what they called bat blindness, and wrote about it in "The Book of the Eyes." Perhaps what they were treating was actually RP.

An often-cited study from over two decades ago of more than six hundred people with RP found that in those who started out with milder disease, taking higher amounts of vitamin A decreased the rate of progression of visual field loss and slowed the deterioration of photoreceptors (as measured by the electroretinogram test). This study is important because it is one of the largest pieces we've found so far of the puzzle of how to treat RP—yet there are so many other missing puzzle pieces.

Because liver is overloaded with many other vitamins, it may not be the best way to get your vitamin A. Better sources include all the carotenoid-rich foods we've discussed so far, along with salmon and trout, which brings us back to the omega-3 oils and DHA. A recent study showed that a vitamin A–rich diet with omega-3 fatty acids decreased the rate of loss of vision—specifically visual acuity, or the sharpness of vision as judged by the ability to read—in RP. Another study showed that adding lutein to the vitamin A slowed down the rate of loss of side vision in RP. And, of course, these nutrients really work in synergy.

WHAT DO BULLS, CURRY, AND MINT HAVE IN COMMON?

Taurine is an amino acid—a protein building block—that was first discovered about two hundred years ago in the gallbladder of bulls, and thus named using the Latin word for bull: taurus. We'll look at taurine again in chapter 7 on diabetes, but it is believed to be helpful as an antioxidant, to stabilize cell membranes, and to regulate fluids within cells. More important for RP, a growing body of evidence suggests that it can help rescue injured neurons in the retina.

78

Taurine, one of the most concentrated protein building blocks in the retina, grabs on to vitamin A and transports it to the photoreceptors in the retina. After vitamin A gets used up by these rods and cones, taurine picks up the spent vitamin A and takes it out for recycling.

One of the main spices in curry powder is turmeric, which comes from the ginger-like root of a native Indian plant and gives it its yellow color. Turmeric contains a biologically active component called curcumin and other curcuminoids (curcumin-like molecules), powerful antioxidants with anti-inflammatory activities, particularly in neural tissue such as the retina. It can also activate genes within cells. Research has shown that curcumin can protect against RP in rats who had the gene defect but not full-blown RP.

And third, the unique mint, *coleus forskohlii* (which we'll talk about much more in chapter 8 on glaucoma), can increase production of a signaling molecule within the retina called cyclic AMP (or cAMP for short) that helps protect and promote survival of neural cells—and in RP, we want these photoreceptors to survive despite having the gene defect. While it is difficult to find this specific mint in your local grocer's produce section, you may find herbal supplements that contain extracts from this mint, or alternatively other fresh mints may have similar benefits.

COENZYME Q10: IS IT EVERYWHERE?

Coenzyme Q10—or Q10 for short (also called vitamin Q and ubiquinone, short for ubiquitous quinone) is a compound that is everywhere you need energy. It helps the power plants within our cells—the mitochondria—produce energy through a process of taking electrons (negatively charged particles) and transferring protons (positively charged particles) to create a gradient, similar to how batteries and fuel cells transmit energy. This is why athletes often use Q10 to enhance performance. Because the retina is the most metabolically active tissue in our bodies, Q10 plays an essential role.

Q10 has other vision-preserving functions. In a similar manner to how it transfers protons in the power plants of our cells, within the retina Q10 transfers protons in the trash incinerators in our cells, called lysosomes, which digest the debris produced by the retina. Protons that accumulate within the lysosomes make these trash incinerators more acidic so that they can more effectively digest that debris.

When light hits the retina, it triggers its typical chain reaction chemical cascade that results in a signal being eventually sent to the brain. But this chemical cascade produces excess electrons— that, if not removed, attack oxygen within the cells. When oxygen is attacked, it forms a powerful oxidant called superoxide, which does what any oxidant does: steals electrons and causes damage. Q10 is a powerful antioxidant that also acts as an "electron sink" or a "mini capacitor"—meaning it can vacuum up all these excess electrons. All this is believed to help with retinal disease, such as RP and macular degeneration, and with glaucoma and cataracts. In addition, it can boost the immune defense system, protect against cancer, decrease atherosclerosis, slow down the progression of Alzheimer's disease, and prevent migraines.

Meats and fish as well as walnuts, pistachios, peanuts, hazelnuts, and almonds are the best sources of Q10. Milk is also a good source. The one best source is green beans! The other vegetables contain quite a bit less Q10, but the ones to go for include spinach, broccoli, sweet potatoes, green peppers, and carrots. Too much Q10 can cause headaches, fatigue, rashes, and gastrointestinal symptoms such as upset stomach or nausea. While it can also lower blood sugars, too much Q10 can cause dangerously low blood sugars as well as dangerously low blood pressure. Natural foods will often give you good amounts without going overboard.

SUMMARY 6: RETINITIS PIGMENTOSA

Retinitis pigmentosa (RP) is a retinal condition that starts in childhood and consists of progressive decline in side vision and inability to see in the dark.

RP is a neurodegeneration of the retina that is dictated by genetic defects that result in a slow loss of rods then cones.

Despite our knowledge of defects in nearly two hundred genes that cause RP, there are no cures or effective medical interventions, other than nutrition.

Retinal cells are made of more than 70 percent fat, so that their membranes can remain "liquidy" to allow light-sensing pigments and other components to flow freely and quickly.

There are two types of essential (because we need them from our diets) fatty acids: omega-3 and omega-6 oils.

Important nutrients from chapter 6:

- DHA—a special type of omega-3 oil that is concentrated in the retina.

- Carotenoids—powerful antioxidants including beta-carotene, lutein, zeaxanthin, astaxanthin (from red marine species), and crocin and crocetin (from saffron).

- Vitamin A—required for the light-sensing pigment in photoreceptors.

- Taurine—an amino acid that transports vitamin A to the retina and then takes it out for recycling.

- Curcumin and curcuminoids—the active components of turmeric in curry powder are powerful antioxidants.

- *Coleus forskohlii*—a mint that promotes survival of neural cells.

- Coenzyme Q10—a compound that is essential for energy production and debris digestion.

CHAPTER 7

DIABETES AND YOUR VISION: A FOCUS ON DIABETIC RETINOPATHY AND MACULAR EDEMA

It's five o'clock on a weekday. For most of us who work, the bell rings, and we're out the door. (Well, some of us have to keep working longer hours.) But for the most part, many people hop in their cars and enter the phenomenon of rush hour bumper-to-bumper traffic. It settles down as cars make it home one-by-one, drivers and passengers ready to take off their shoes and grab a bite to eat.

Well imagine a part of the country where a new law requires that no car park on the street or in any driveway. All cars must park either in a garage or in a community parking lot, and all these community parking lots are gated. At the end of the day, you'll see some cars driving around, but most cars will be either inside a garage or in a community parking lot. But what if there suddenly was a shortage of garage door opener batteries and all the existing batteries started to die all at once, or the ticket machines or card swipes at the parking lot gates started to malfunction? People couldn't get into their garages or into their community parking lots, but because they're not allowed to park on the streets or driveways, they'd have to keep driving and driving. Some cars would run out of gas, some might break down, and rush hour traffic would keep going on and on. What a mess it would be.

Let's turn to diabetes—and then come back to this parking mess. The meals we eat contain different types of carbohydrates, which is the chemical word for sugars. These range from the commonly recognized simple sugars (like table sugar or sucrose) to fruit sugars (fructose) to milk sugars (lactose) to complex sugars such as those in breads, pastas, and cereals. Sugars are everywhere! These sugars are essential for our bodies, providing our cells with energy and ways of storing that energy; forming components of enzyme "helper molecules" within our cells; even forming fundamental parts of our genetic material (think DNA) within our cells. While the big role of sugars is providing energy to our cells, sugars play key roles in many cell functions, from our immune system to disease prevention.

When we eat a meal, our digestive system processes the foods and sends the sugars from our foods into our bloodstream. They swim around our bloodstream heading for a cell that needs some sugar. Well, all our cells need sugars; sugars are essential for our bodies. However, when we eat, the floodgates open up and the sugars just pour into our bloodstream. And much of that sugar needs to be directed toward storage sites, for later use, or high-energy sites that need the sugars right away. The storage sites are adipose cells (commonly called fat cells) and liver cells, and the high-energy sites are muscle and heart cells. Muscle cells also double-up as storage sites; they are able to store sugars for later use as well. These storage and high-energy sites account for two-thirds of all of our cells in our bodies (and a recent study estimated that we have about thirty-seven trillion cells in our bodies . . . that's a lot of cells).

INSULIN

So our bodies have a system to control the flow of sugars into these storage and high-energy cells, which involves a hormone called insulin. Insulin controls the body's flow of sugars into most (but not all) of our cells. When there's a lot of sugar in the bloodstream, insulin opens gates in the storage and high-energy sites, the parking lots and garages.

But insulin does much more than that. To say that insulin controls blood sugars is like declaring that Ben Franklin was a Founding Father of the United States and stopping there. Yes, he was, but he was also an inventor (of bifocal glasses, among other things), scientist (experiments on flying a kite in a lightning storm—never try at home!), author (*Poor Richard's Almanac*), politician, postmaster, and much more.

Insulin also controls processes in our cells that involve the use of sugars. Because sugars form components of enzyme "helper molecules," insulin increases the activity of enzymes. Because sugars form key parts of our DNA, insulin also increases DNA production activities and the use of DNA for making proteins. Insulin helps cells grow. It controls some of the electrolytes, such as potassium, magnesium, and phosphate in our bodies. We are learning that insulin plays an important role in inflammation and also affects how our brains function; interestingly it is an essential component of good memory and learning, helping the synaptic connections that develop during memory formation. Perhaps that's why it's hard to forget that chicken salad that made us sick six months ago—neuropsychologists have suggested this connection between foods and memory exists to help us remember foods to avoid.

We now know how important insulin really is. So what happens when our body stops making insulin (which is what happens in type 1 diabetes) or when the body either makes some but not enough insulin or doesn't properly sense it (which is what happens in type 2 diabetes)? Well, we will then have problems with enzyme "helper molecules," with DNA production, with growth of cells, with electrolytes, with memory, and a whole host of biological issues. But most important, we'll have trouble regulating the sugar in our bodies. Now let's get back to that rush hour traffic.

INSULIN PREVENTS THE SUGAR TRAFFIC JAM THE BLOODSTREAM

What happens when there is no control of the flow of sugars into storage and high-energy cells? It's just like what happens in our rush hour traffic scenario when the garage door openers don't work and the ticket machines or card swipes malfunction. All the cars get stuck driving around the streets, breaking down at times, but really causing a lot of congestion and a seemingly never-ending rush hour. After we eat a meal, the sugars that enter our bloodstream swim around looking for that garage or parking lot—the storage sites and high-energy sites. Insulin opens the door and lets them into those sites. But if there's no insulin to open the gates or if the gates are not sensitive to the insulin, then the sugars keep swimming around in the bloodstream, seemingly endlessly, until they get broken down, and until they break down the cells that make the walls of the blood vessels. This damage to the walls of blood vessels eventually wreaks havoc on the eyes, causing blood vessels to leak and bleed, and causes decreased blood flow to tissue.

MACULAR EDEMA

Let's start with blood vessel leaking. Think of your front lawn, or better yet, if your front lawn is anything like mine, perhaps think about your neighbor's perfect green immaculate lawn that they're constantly watering with a sprinkler. Well if that hose starts to get damaged over the years, it starts to spring leaks that cause areas of the lawn to get soggy. If you don't dry up these soggy areas, the green grass starts to die and you end up with muddy patches. The same thing happens in the retina. Over years of having excess sugars swimming in your bloodstream, the blood vessels start to get damaged and start to spring leaks. These leaks cause sogginess in the retina. This sogginess we call edema, specifically diabetic macular edema, when it is caused by diabetes and affects the center of the retina (the macula). The fluid buildup in the retina often causes decreased vision. Our main solution is to seal up the leaking blood vessels, but if the blood sugars remain high, then you'll often spring more leaks, and we're just running around in circles. That's why we need to stop the cycle. Proper nutrition is often an essential component of stopping that cycle.

DIABETIC RETINOPATHY

But diabetes doesn't just cause sogginess: It can decrease blood flow in the retina. Often, diabetes is accompanied by high blood pressure (or hypertension). If the pressure through the water system is too high, because you've turned the water spigot up too high, then to control the amount of water that comes out of the sprinkler, the flow through the hose has to be decreased. The body has a way to do this: The blood vessels start to narrow over time, so that the lumen of the blood vessels gets thinner. So now you have thinner, more fragile blood vessels, more prone to springing leaks.

The sugars swimming in the bloodstream also cause spots of partial blockage; if the water is full of "crud," then that grime starts to accumulate on the inside of the hose, damaging it and causing less water to flow out to the lawn. Blocked blood vessels from retinopathy cause balloon-like dilatations to form—similar to what happens in a blocked garden hose with the water turned up all the way. These ballooned areas develop tiny leaks and suddenly the lawn is soggy in that area. And vision blurs.

In addition, blood flow becomes limited in areas of the retina— which, remember, requires high blood flow. You can imagine what happens if blood flow is decreased. If your neighbor's beautiful lawn has a water-thirsty type of grass that requires a lot of watering, then

86

a little less watering would start to create yellow spots, or patches where the grass starts to die off. When parts of the retina get starved of blood supply and the oxygen and nutrients that come with proper blood supply, these parts of the retina start to slowly die off. If it involves the center of the retina, then vision is affected. Unlike grass, when retina cells are lost, they can't be replaced. When it affects the center of the retina (the macula), which is the center of our vision, we call this process macular ischemia (lack of blood flow). Proper nutrition can help us prevent getting to that point.

In severe cases of diabetic retinopathy (the retinal injury from diabetes), the blocked flow causes the body to build new blood vessels. In theory this sounds good, except that these new vessels grow uncontrolled like weeds and damage the retina. It's like waking up one day and suddenly noticing that you've forgotten to water your front lawn for the past few months (or that the watering of the front lawn has been spotty and ineffective). You run to your garage and search for whatever additional hose that you have to try to supplement the watering. You find some old ratty hose in the corner of the garage that's been sitting there for years. You can't even untangle the hose, you just connect it to your spigot and throw the tangle into your lawn. It's a big mess, a big clump of tangled hose, that doesn't water your lawn very well and leaks. Well, in the retina, in response to the lack of blood supply, these new blood vessels that grow are a big mess just like that tangled hose. They don't nourish the retina very well at all, they leak fluid, they bleed, and they block vision. We call this proliferative diabetic retinopathy, because of the proliferation of these new blood vessels.

If you're so desperate to water your lawn and the first tangled clump of ratty hose doesn't work, you may run back to your garage and get another tangled clump of old hose and just toss it out onto your lawn. When that doesn't work, you may get more tangled clumps and throw them out. Suddenly, your lawn is full of all these tangled clumps of hose. Well, a retina could not function properly at all that way. These uncontrolled new blood vessels start to stick to the retina and as they grow, they pull on the retina, causing the retina to distort or even detach from its position. It's like someone pulling your wallpaper off your walls, causing the wallpaper to tent up in areas, or even tear. When the retina tents up in areas, we call that a retinal detachment. When the retina tears, you run the risk of the entire retina falling out of position, like wallpaper falling off the wall.

Not surprisingly, uncontrolled blood vessel development can ravage the retina and your vision, and it is often very difficult to treat. Fortunately, most diabetic retinopathy is treatable, manageable, and often can even be prevented (more so with type 2 diabetes) with changes in diet and lifestyle—along with medications—before the symptoms truly take hold. Typically, diabetes-related eye conditions only happen after years of poor blood sugar control (or, in other words, the patient not treating his or her diabetes). Once the diabetes is treated, most vision problems resolve themselves if caught early enough, including diabetic macular edema and proliferative diabetic retinopathy.

DIABETES, CATARACTS, AND DRY EYE

Two other important common ways that diabetes leads to vision loss are cataracts (which we learn more about in chapter 9) and dry eye (which we learn more about in chapter 10). As an introduction to the topic, though, let's touch on how diabetes causes these two conditions. Diabetes has been estimated to cause a five-times increased risk of developing cataracts. Diabetes causes poor blood supply and poor nutrition to the lens. It also causes the buildup of toxic proteins called advanced glycation end products, also known as AGEs. Excess sugars in the body start to bind to proteins (a process called glycation) causing these proteins to become toxic. In diabetes, these toxic proteins—these AGEs—further exacerbate the leakiness of blood vessels; they cause inflammation and they cause oxidation. When we delve into these mechanisms, we start to see how much overlap there is between various types of injuries on a cellular level. In the lens in the eye, all these types of injuries cause the lens to be cloudy and a cataract to form.

We'll leave the rest of the discussion of cataracts to chapter 9, but let's briefly also talk about the cornea and dry eye. Just as diabetes damages the retina, diabetes damages nerve fibers throughout the body. You may have heard of diabetic neuropathy, which means diabetic damage to nerves. Nerve fibers depend on blood supply and blood vessels for nourishment. So as diabetes affects blood vessels, it affects blood supply to nerves. Remember, the cornea has more sensory nerve endings per square millimeter than anywhere else in the body, which is why it hurts so much to get even a speck of dust in the eye. Well, as diabetes damages nerves in the cornea, the nerve fibers start to lose their ability to function and don't provide the proper sensation to the cornea so that it turns on the windshield wipers (eyelids) or the washer fluid / lubricant (tears), and the cornea starts to dry out. We'll talk more about dry eye in chapter 10, but it is important to know that diabetes has a profound effect on nerves in the eye, particularly the nerves that control the surface of the eye.

BEYOND THE EYES

In fact diabetes causes a lot of problems throughout the whole body, not just in the eyes, but in the heart, kidney, brain, and elsewhere. So what does someone with diabetes feel? Sometimes there are no symptoms of diabetes. Other times, the symptoms may be fairly mild, such as increased thirstiness or increased hunger. You may feel fatigued, and sometimes the fatigue can be quite severe.

Nerve damage to the hands or feet can cause numbness or tingling. Sores that develop may not heal properly or even heal at all. And, of course, blurred vision, blocked vision, and loss of vision are frequent manifestations.

Many health researchers now consider diabetes to be an epidemic due to increasing obesity and broad consumption of processed and fast foods. Over twenty-five million people in the United States have diabetes—that's one out of every twelve Americans—and that number is on the rise: Seventy-nine million people have tested as pre-diabetic, meaning that, without substantial change, they will one day be diagnosed with full-blown diabetes. All diabetics are at risk for either diabetic retinopathy or macular edema—and nearly half of the diabetics in the United States have those eye problems today—but one-third are unaware of their illness.

What we see in the eye occurs throughout the body. For example, diabetes is the number one cause of heart disease in the United States. The small blood vessel changes in the heart often precede the onset of detectable heart disease in diabetes, and this shows up in your eyes. In other words, there are no early markers available to detect small blood vessel heart disease in diabetes, no blood test, no urine test, no EKG or heart test—except for an eye exam. The same thing can be generally applied to the rest of the body: Blood vessel changes in the eye mirror what occurs throughout the body in diabetes. Unfortunately, the vast majority of diabetic patients do not seek eye care until visual symptoms begin.

TREATMENT THROUGH NUTRITION

Like diabetic retinopathy, diabetic changes throughout the body can be managed and treated through proper healthy nutrition, along with a regimen that often includes exercise and medication—with type 1 diabetes replacement for the body's missing insulin is an absolute requirement, while with type 2 diabetes some patients are able to control their diabetes without medication. The most important treatment for diabetes is controlling blood sugars, often by limiting the amount of sugars eaten, along with the use of insulin and other medications as appropriate. Keeping blood vessels in tip-top shape includes making sure blood pressure is controlled and ensuring blood cholesterol levels are not high so that cholesterol doesn't cause further damage to the blood vessels.

You may hear reports of very discouraging data on nutrition and diabetic retinopathy. In one example, a recent large analysis of over four thousand people involved in fifteen separate studies showed no association between diabetic retinopathy and diet or blood levels of specific nutrients. But this doesn't mean that nutrients don't help in diabetes. Managing diabetes starts with good nutrition. It's a team approach, involving your family doctor or internist and other medical specialists, and making sure that you keep your body healthy and keep sugar intake down. You can never eliminate all the sugars from your diet, nor should you, so good balanced nutrition is essential.

We've discussed alpha-lipoic acid, the "antioxidant of antioxidants"—an essential soldier in the war against oxidation that helps prevent the toxic oxidation effects of AGEs and may actually block AGEs from forming in the first place. Alpha-lipoic acid may also enhance sensitivity to insulin through insulin-signaling pathways inside of cells, and enhance the role of insulin in transporting sugars and redistributing sugar transporters to where they are needed the most. As such, it helps control the sugar levels in the blood. Numerous studies show that alpha-lipoic acid can help with decreasing retinopathy in animals. Until there are the same studies in humans, we can simply assume that diabetics who take alpha-lipoic acid will also have less oxidative stress and oxidative damage in their bloodstream.

Remember, getting your daily dose of antioxidants is so important, and not just for diabetes.

Importance of Bioflavonoids in Diabetes

The bioflavonoids we talked about in chapter 1 have been shown to improve capillary (small blood vessel) health in diabetes. One of the most active bioflavonoids is quercetin, a plant-derived ring-shaped nutrient. It's a powerful antioxidant. More than that, scientific evidence suggests that it blocks the pathway that forms toxic AGEs in diabetes, thereby decreasing the damaging effects of high blood sugars. It also may inhibit the formation of the new blood vessel growth. These effects are not only important for diabetes, but for many other eye conditions, such as macular degeneration which we learned about in chapter 5, and for eye health in general. Quercetin may be beneficial in preventing or protecting against macular degeneration, cataracts, inflammation in the eye, pink eye, and other eye conditions. To get your daily quercetin, go for the hot chile peppers. Other wise choices include red onions, black-eyed peas, and okra. Bee pollen is also quite high in quercetin.

Troxerutin. So while we're on a roll with plants, let's talk about troxerutin, a bioflavonoid that comes from the Japanese pagoda tree. It's a particularly active derivative of the bioflavonoid rutin, which can also be processed into quercetin, the powerful bioflavonoid about which we just learned. I've gone through the files at Johns Hopkins and found records from back in the 1940s of research on the benefits of rutin for retinal blood vessels and disease of the retinal veins. A small clinical trial from a couple of decades ago demonstrated that troxerutin improved vision in patients who suffered from a blood clot in their retinal vein—called a retinal vein occlusion. Troxerutin improved vision, improved retinal blood vessel circulation, and decreased fluid buildup in the retina. These are the same processes with which we need help in diabetes. You can find rutin in citrus fruit, apples (particularly the peels), peaches, apricots, cranberries, asparagus, green peppers, and one of the best sources for rutin: buckwheat.

Resveratrol. Resveratrol, another bioflavonoid, was first discovered by Japanese researcher Michio Takaoka, many decades ago, in the 1930s, but has been touted only recently for its ability to extend life, after discovery that it prolonged the lifespan of worms and some types of fish. It has been found to dramatically activate an anti-aging gene—also found in humans—that's involved in repairing damaged DNA and making mitochondria (the power stations of cells), controlling inflammation, and regulating insulin secretion. Though there's not enough strong scientific data to support its anti-aging effects in humans at this point, there's enough data to support its health benefits, through its antioxidant and anti-cancer activities, which certainly would help you live a healthier life and perhaps longer. It can help protect against macular degeneration, and, similar to quercetin, may inhibit the formation of new blood vessel growth.

Resveratrol is a plant "phytochemical" that protects plants from invading bacteria or mold by attacking the invaders. However, unlike other bioflavonoids and unlike quercetin, the natural sources of resveratrol are limited, particularly to the skin of grapes, particularly muscadine grapes. So many people seek it in wines, but there's a lot of conflicting data about wines and there are researchers who caution against seeking bioflavonoids in wines because of other harmful effects . . . it may be best to seek these bioflavonoids in fruits and vegetables in their natural states. And, keep in mind that there are thousands of different types of bioflavonoids and many we don't even know about: For diabetes, go for the vegetables in their natural states.

Three Metals and a Metalloid That Help in Diabetes

Although you may remember the part in chapter 1 about metals causing oxidation and rust, you may also remember the "good" metals we talked about: manganese and magnesium. The themes and nutrients in this book keep coming around over and over again, because they are so intertwined. The human body is, of course, one body, composed of multiple types of tissues. So what helps one part of the body is likely to help another part of the body. Four examples follow.

Magnesium. Magnesium is believed to help with the body's ability to properly move and use sugars. As such, it may play an essential role in preventing diabetes. It also helps regulate blood flow through blood vessels by releasing nitric oxide, a signaling molecule that helps blood vessels dilate. Nitric oxide is such an important blood vessel regulator that three scientists (Robert Furchgott, Louis Ignarro, and Ferid Murad) won the 1998 Nobel Prize for this discovery. Just keep in mind that nitric oxide is not the same as nitrous oxide (laughing gas at the dentist). As a side note, nitric oxide also helps prevent infections, particularly in our sinuses, lungs, and throats, and helps prevent against osteoporosis by blocking cells that eat bone. For the eye, magnesium helps regulate nitric oxide, which may prevent high blood pressure and maintain proper blood flow in the retina, particularly in diabetes.

Chromium. Chromium is the metal that makes the beautiful chrome plating on motorcycles and older cars. We've discussed how chromium can help remove the drusen that forms behind the retina in macular degeneration. Scientists believe that it plays an important role in helping diabetics by regulating sugar use by cells, and it works in close conjunction with insulin, regulating insulin and blood sugars. It may also help with cholesterol levels in the body. Keep in mind, though, that 99 percent of the chromium you eat gets excreted by your digestive system. It never makes it into your bloodstream. That's probably helpful, as you don't want to get too much chromium. And, don't worry, the chromium that you eat (called trivalent chromium—having three electrons) is a different form from the chromium (hexavalent chromium—with six electrons) that poisoned the town's drinking water in the movie *Erin Brockovich*. (Hexavalent chromium causes skin and eye irritation and just half a teaspoon can be lethal.)

Vanadium. Metals can indeed cause oxidative damage. Vanadium is no exception. Through oxidative damage, it can cause breaks in our DNA and interfere with enzymes that produce energy in our cells. It can be particularly toxic throughout our eyes, as well as throughout the body. However, there has been excitement in the past about vanadium. Why? By mimicking the action of insulin or improving the body's sensitivity to insulin, it may help decrease blood sugars in diabetics. There is also some limited evidence that it may decrease blood pressure and perhaps lower cholesterol. Athletes often use it to enhance their performance. It's likely that just a small amount of vanadium is probably all we need, and we certainly shouldn't overdo it. Just like chromium, vanadium (originally called panchromium) has a hard time getting absorbed by our bodies—for a good reason—and so most of it is excreted. You'll get all the vanadium you need through seafood, such as lobster; nuts, such as hazelnuts or pecans; beans, such as lentils, green peas, and navy beans; and vegetables, such as alfalfa, radishes, cabbage, parsley, turnip greens, potatoes, and squash.

Boron. A metalloid? Yes, this sometimes is found as a metal, but other times just a powder. Borax, the cleaner, comes from boron. There's even a town within the Mojave Desert in California named Boron after the boron mines there. Within our bodies, boron helps enhance enzyme activity and the availability of hormones, helping maintain proper hormonal balance in both men and women. This proper hormonal balance in turn supports bone health and, for the eye, it balances cholesterol levels, decreases inflammation, and there is evidence that it helps regulate blood sugars. In fact, in the retina, through its hormonal-mediated ability to raise the good cholesterol—HDL—boron indirectly helps get more nutrients to the retina, specifically lutein and zeaxanthin (the natural sunglasses we learned about in chapter 5) as they hitch a ride with the HDL that transports them there. Some of the best natural sources for boron are peanuts, black-eyed peas, lima beans, onions, broccoli, carrots, peaches, grapes, apples, and pears.

Proteins Make You Strong, And . . .

A friend I'll call Richard came to me one day. After about eight years of diabetes, he was having a hard time controlling his blood sugars. Richard was a do-it-yourselfer who thought he could just do everything on his own, including treating his diabetes. He'd tried cutting back as much as possible on dietary sugars, and then he read about how proteins can help diabetics. He bought vegetable protein powder at his local nutrition store and started mixing it in with everything he ate and even everything he drank. It made everything more than just a bit chalky tasting, but Richard swore by it. He was taking in a ton of protein each day, but he forgot that excess proteins get broken down in the body and converted to . . . yes, sugar! So his bloodstream was just getting overloaded with sugar converted from proteins. Once again, the theme of too much of a good thing arises. Keep in mind that excess proteins can also cause dehydration, stress the kidneys, and cause loss of calcium, which can weaken bones. In someone with pre-existing liver disease or kidney disease (which many diabetics have), excess proteins can also cause a buildup of ammonia in the body, resulting in serious illness. When Richard cut back on the proteins, his blood sugars normalized and were under control again. On the other end of the extreme, that doesn't mean that diabetics should skip the proteins.

There is a definite role for them. Here are two helpful nutrients from proteins:

Taurine. As previously discussed, taurine, the amino-acid, protein building block, works in our gallbladders to regulate the amount of cholesterol that we absorb in our diets. As such, taurine is very helpful for diabetics. This protein also acts as an antioxidant, though not a strong one, and can help decrease levels of the blood vessel–damaging toxin homocysteine. By reducing inflammation and decreasing blood pressure, taurine benefits anyone who has diabetes or wants to protect against diabetes. Most important, since the 1930s studies on taurine have suggested that it may help lower blood sugar. While it is uncertain how or if taurine interacts with insulin, it certainly helps diabetics. Through its effects, it may prevent AGEs from forming and stabilize leaky cells to decrease swelling or edema. You can get your taurine through meats, particularly flounder, and through dairy products (milk). Seaweed is a very good vegetable source of taurine!

Carnitine. We learned about the drusen buster carnitine— formed from amino acids—in chapter 5. Originally known as vitamin BT, carnitine is neither a vitamin nor an essential nutrient. But it is essentially helpful! In diabetes, carnitine has been shown to decrease the formation of the AGEs produced when the sugars attack proteins. It has been suggested to be particularly helpful in preventing diabetic cataracts. It's found in meats, and to a lesser extent in fish and dairy products.

But remember what we learned from Richard, and let's keep a balanced approach. And as any diabetic knows, let's not forget to focus on limiting sugars, particularly artificial sugars. Sugar is everywhere, and our bodies have a natural attraction to sugar.

SUMMARY 7: DIABETES AND YOUR VISION

Sugars come in many forms and provide our bodies with energy, form components of "helper molecules" within our cells, and form key parts of our genetic material (DNA).

Insulin is a hormone that controls the flow of sugars into our cells and many more functions, such as increasing activity of enzymes, increasing DNA production, helping cells grow, controlling electrolytes, and even supporting healthy brain function.

When there is little or no insulin to control the flow of sugars into our cells, excess sugars remain swimming in our bloodstream, causing damage to the blood vessels.

Diabetes also causes toxic proteins called advanced glycation end products—AGEs—that cause further damage to the eye and body.

Diabetic macular edema is swelling in the retina caused by damaged leaky blood vessels, often resulting in decreased vision.

Proliferative diabetic retinopathy is caused by a proliferation of new blood vessels in response to decreased blood flow from sugar-damaged blood vessels.

Important nutrients from chapter 7:

- Alpha-lipoic acid—prevents effects of AGEs and enhances sensitivity to insulin.
- Quercetin—a bioflavonoid that is a powerful antioxidant.
- Troxerutin—a bioflavonoid that is beneficial for retinal blood vessels.
- Resveratrol—a bioflavonoid that activates an anti-aging gene involved in regulating insulin secretion.
- Magnesium—a metal that helps the body properly move and use sugars and regulate blood flow.

- Chromium—a metal that regulates insulin and blood sugars.

- Vanadium—a potentially toxic metal that improves the body's sensitivity to insulin.

- Boron—a metalloid that helps enzyme activity and enhances the availability of hormones.

- Taurine—an amino acid that is an antioxidant and decreases the toxin homocysteine.

- Carnitine—formed from amino acids, it decreases the formation of AGEs.

CHAPTER 8
GLAUCOMA: SILENT SUFFERERS

In one of my favorite cities, New York City, urban legend has it that there are a dozen rats for every human being. That's millions of rats. Author Robert Sullivan was inspired to write about the lives of these swarming vermin after being moved by a painting of rats by the naturalist artist and ornithologist John Audubon, after whom the Audubon Society was founded. (In an ironic twist, Audubon found, returning home to Kentucky after an extended time away, that rats had eaten hundreds of his drawings of birds stored in a wooden box.) Most of us are oblivious to the presence of rats in our cities, even as they are chewing away at the wiring and electric cables below the buildings, as if these wires and cables were Twizzlers.

Glaucoma is a slow loss of signal connection—a neurologic disorder—of the optic nerve that sends the images the retina forms to the brain. Well, perhaps a rat starts chewing on this wiring—this optic nerve—without anyone knowing. Just like the rats below New York City chew on wires without us knowing, without any side effects, the optic nerve still sends signals to the brain even as it is chewed, tattered, and torn. You won't notice what's going on until one day when the nibbles get so extensive that the signal is weak or lost. That's when you'll know you have glaucoma.

As an eye doctor, I look at the back of the eye and assess the health of this nerve. We see it in cross-section. So imagine a thick electric cord or cable wire that is cut off on one end as it inserts into the eyeball—that's what we see. We can't see its sides, so we have to assess the nerve by just looking at its end. This cable or cord—the optic nerve—is a bundle of 1.2 million individual fibers that we could never count even if we tried. So when we look at it on-end, we apply our training as an eye doctor to evaluate its over-all health.

Glaucoma is the neurologic disorder characterized by the loss of these nerve fibers. With the rats nibbling at the side of the wiring, the wire sometimes becomes thinner. So when rats chew away some of those 1.2 million fibers, we see what appears to be fewer fibers in the cross-sectional end of the nerve as it inserts into the eyeball. Sometime we can definitively identify fewer fibers, just by looking, but many times we only have a suspicion that there are fewer. Today, new imaging helps us tell if there are fewer nerve fibers.

In the early stages of glaucoma, when the rats have only done some very mild nibbling, there will often be no noticeable changes in one's vision. But detailed testing of the visual field (the ability to see the full picture, including all the sides and edges of the picture as well as the center of the picture) will often show some subtle blind spots at the edges of the picture, the edges of the visual field. The gnawing at the edges of the wiring often spares the center until very late in the process.

In the case of glaucoma, the process of nibbling takes years if not decades. Some subtle blind spots may appear early along the sides of the visual field, but these are only detectable by the eye doctor. We really don't pay much attention to our side vision in day-to-day activity, and these subtle blind spots will certainly go unnoticed as our brains find ways to fill them in. We all know about the larger blind spot we all have in our vision, just to the right of center in our right eye and to the left of center in our left eye. Pick a spot in front of you about two feet away. Close one eye and look directly at that spot. Take a yellow pencil with a red eraser and hold the red eraser right at that spot at about arm's length. Move the red eraser slowly to the right (if you're testing your right eye) but keep look-ing straight at the spot and not the eraser as it moves, and after a few inches the red eraser will disappear into our natural blind spot, which is where the optic nerve connects to the retina.

Glaucoma is a disorder that can strike at any age, although it usually is diagnosed in older people. It can permanently damage vision and is the second leading cause of blindness in the world. Over time, side vision is lost and as that progresses, the loss creeps slowly and gradually inward, forming tunnel vision. Symptoms tend to reveal themselves once the damage has been done and the disease is quite advanced.

With glaucoma, several different kinds of figurative rats gnaw away at the optic nerve between the eye and the brain. The most common "rat" is high pressure in the eye. When many people think of glaucoma, they think of high pressure, and they think that high pressure is glaucoma. High pressure is not glaucoma; rather, it's a serious risk factor for glaucoma, just like having an over-inflated basketball or car tire. Over time, the pressure pushes against the optic nerve and the cells that make up the optic nerve, slowly causing the cells and the fibers—the wiring—to start to tatter away, causing glaucoma. Maintaining proper fluid balance in the eye is essential.

PRESSURE IN THE EYE AS A RISK FACTOR

What causes the pressure in the eye to go up? Let's start with what causes a bathtub to overflow. To maintain a full bathtub without it overflowing, you either adjust the flow of water or the position of the stopper in the drain. If you keep the stopper plugging the drain, and you keep the water on (whether the water is on high or on a low flow), then the bathtub will overflow. If you pull the stopper out part-way but the water is on too high, the bathtub may still overflow.

The eye works similarly. There is a part of the eye, inside the eye, behind the iris (the colored part of the eye) that produces fluid that fills up the inside hollow part of the eye. Let's call that tissue the faucet. There is also a drain in front of the iris, all along the edge where the iris meets the white part of the eye from the inside. This drain is called the trabecular meshwork. When it gets clogged, the pressure in the eye goes up. Likewise when the faucet is turned up too high, even if the drain is not clogged, the pressure in the eye goes up. Treatment for eye pressure (which we call intraocular pressure) is aimed at turning the faucet down—usually through medications—or increasing the drainage, either by using medications or with surgery to create new drains in the bathtub.

OTHER RISK FACTORS FOR GLAUCOMA

There are other risk factors (think rats) for glaucoma, not just eye pressure. Blood flow to the optic nerve is believed to play an important role, and just like we learned in chapter 3, proper blood flow is essential for good eye health. Oxidative damage (discussed in chapter 1) also plays a central role, though scientists are still trying to tease out how. Perhaps even inflammation and loss of proper scaffolding support for the optic nerve also lead to development of glaucoma. In all these cases, proper nutrition is important for keeping the eye in shape to prevent glaucoma or, if it's already in process, to protect against further nerve injury. Perhaps real rats enjoy fruits and vegetables, but the rats in glaucoma certainly don't!

The good news is that if glaucoma is detected early enough, it's possible to slow the progress of the disease medically and nutritionally.

VITAMIN B1, THE ORIGINAL "VITAL AMINE"

Let's start with the original "vit-amine," vitamin B1. The Polish biochemist Dr. Kazimierz Funk characterized the compound as an "amine" type (meaning it contains nitrogen), as well as noting how vital it was for life—a vital amine, or vit-amine for short. Dutch physician Dr. Christiaan Eijkman was actually the first to discover the substance we now call vitamin B1, and he went on to win a Nobel Prize for his discovery of vitamins. He did this by observing that there was some substance in rice, which we now know is vitamin B1, which prevented a disease called beri-beri, also known as endemic neuritis. This neurologic disorder is characterized by damage to the nerves in the hands and legs, resulting in pain, tingling, weakness, and eventually an inability to walk—hence the Sri Lankan word "beri-beri," which means weakness and is literally translated as "I can't, I can't."

Vitamin B1 is essential in the pathway that makes the body's energy packets—called ATP. For cells to function, they need energy, and they don't take unleaded gasoline, nor do they take AAA batteries. They take ATP, which the power stations in the cells create on their own from the foods we eat, along with oxygen. So for the optic nerve, vitamin B1 is essential so that the nerve has proper energy—of course the same goes for other high-energy-demanding tissues such as the retina. But much more than energy provision, vitamin B1 is what we call a "neuro-protectant," as it protects neural cells from injury caused by excess release of neurotransmitters, the signals that send messages from one neuronal synapse to another. It also regulates the charged particles that form the impulse signals that get sent through the neuronal axons—the nerve fibers. While vitamin B1 doesn't change the pressure in the eye, it helps protect against the other possible rats that cause glaucoma. A recent study of several thousand people showed that higher vitamin B1 levels in your blood decreased the risk of glaucoma by an impressive 50 percent over ten years! Wow.

Nuts, such as pistachios, pecans, and hazelnuts, are loaded with vitamin B1. You can also get your original vit-amine from edamame, navy beans, black beans, and lentils. Vegetable sources include peas, artichokes, and carrot juice. Breads and cereals are often enriched with vitamin B1.

While we're talking about numbered vitamin Bs, let's touch on vitamin B12. We learned quite a bit about it in chapter 4. Two Japanese studies have shown that vitamin B12 can protect against the deterioration of blind spots at peripheral edges of the visual field in glaucoma and perhaps even reverse some blind spots, or at least improve the ability to recognize light signals and images in the peripheral visual field that would otherwise have gone unrecognized and perhaps have been falsely identified as blind spots.

NEUROLOGIC ASSISTANTS FOR GLAUCOMA

Although not technically a vit-amine, choline is an essential amine. Along with vitamin B5, it forms a neural signaling molecule or a neurotransmitter—called acetylcholine. This neurotransmitter protects against over-stimulation of neural cells by other neurotransmitters. Over-stimulation results in a dangerous process called excitotoxicity, which leads to degeneration and death of neural cells. Choline serves as a very important component in the membranes of neural cells, helping them function properly. Choline also decreases the amount of the vessel-damaging toxin called homocysteine that we learned about in chapter 4. New studies have shown that patients with glaucoma often had higher levels of the toxin homocysteine in their blood than similar people who did not have glaucoma.

Research also suggests choline may improve signaling between the eye and the brain through the optic nerve, and it may protect against deterioration of blind spots at the peripheral edge of the visual field and perhaps even reverse some blind spots. The verdict is still out, but preliminary data is promising. Eggs are a wonderful source for choline . . . just one egg per day gives you about half of all the choline you need. Other high sources include peanuts, cashews, steak, cod, and salmon. You can also find choline in walnuts, brussels sprouts, cauliflower, navy beans, and pinto beans.

Peppermint, spearmint, curly mint, chocolate mint . . . there are hundreds of different types of mint. And the mint family also includes many delicious spices: basil, oregano, lavender, and sage, rosemary, and thyme—sorry Simon and Garfunkel but parsley is from a completely different family! Various mints have been used for centuries as herbal remedies for a variety of conditions.

One particular mint, *coleus forskohlii,* also mentioned in chapter 6, is found in the Indian subcontinent. It has been used for centuries, but was recently discovered to have a special effect: It can activate enzymes that turn up production of an important signaling molecule inside of all of our cells. This signaling molecule, called cyclic AMP (or cAMP for short), is so important because many signaling molecules such as hormones and neural signals (neurotransmitters) can't enter inside cells because cells have a protective encapsulating wall. So when these certain neural signals and hormones need to deliver messages to the inside of cells, they relay the information to cAMP for delivery to the appropriate address. Thus as the coleus mint increases production of cAMP, there are more of these cAMP relay messengers just inside the wall of a cell waiting to deliver that important health message. There is developing research to suggest that, through increasing cAMP availability, this mint may decrease eye pressure (by turning down the faucet in the eye that makes the fluid). Furthermore, this mint may also increase the responsiveness of the neural cells of the eye to specific neural signaling molecules—called neurotrophic factors—that help protect and promote survival of neural cells.

SUPPORTING IMPROVED DRAINAGE IN GLAUCOMA

So how do we protect the drain we talked about—the trabecular meshwork—from getting clogged? First, we have to recognize that the drain is much more complex than a bathtub drain, more than just a metal pipe and a rubber stopper. In your eye, the actual drainage pipe is called Schlemm's canal. Covering this drain is the trabecular meshwork filter that helps regulate the amount of fluid drained and filters it. Every couple of hours or less, all the fluid in the eye is filtered out and replaced. While the amount of fluid is very small (not even a tenth of a liquid ounce), the scale of this process is equivalent to filtering out the bathtub and replacing all the fluid with fresh water every couple of hours.

The amazing thing is that this fluid in the eye is more than just water. It has electrolytes and sugars for energy; it has proteins and antibodies to protect the cells in the eye; it even contains high concentrations of nutrients. For example, the level of vitamin C in this liquid is twenty times higher than in the bloodstream, higher than most anywhere in the body (except for the back of the eye, where vitamin C is one hundred times higher than in the bloodstream).

However, the filter can get clogged, resulting in fluid buildup in the eye. We need nutrients that support this delicate tissue. Collagen and hyaluronic acid are two important compounds that are an integral part of the filter. The filter is similar to a cloth towel or a sponge, with numerous pores, but instead of being made of cotton or synthetic materials, it is made of collagen and hyaluronic acid and specialized cells.

Hyaluronic acid is a very long, long chain of specialized sugars that forms part of our connective tissue, the tissue that makes up joints and our skin. It plays an important role in preventing arthritis in joints and wrinkles in our skin as we age. It also helps the trabecular meshwork maintain its shape, preventing it from collapsing and keeping the pores open. In addition, it supports the optic nerve as it meets and joins the eye. Data show that people with glaucoma have less hyaluronic acid in their trabecular meshwork and in their optic nerve junction. While you could eat a lot of hyaluronic acid by eating rooster combs, very little if any hyaluronic acid gets absorbed by the digestive system. Also, it is uncertain if taking a hyaluronic acid precursor—called glucosamine—is sufficient or helpful in increasing hyaluronic acid levels. The best way may be to eat nutritious foods that contain the nutrients needed to make and stabilize hyaluronic acids: manganese, boron, and bioflavonoids (all of which we learned about in other chapters). Manganese, for example, helps the enzymes that create the components of the hyaluronic acid scaffolding of the optic nerve and trabecular meshwork.

Similarly, collagen is essential to supporting these structures, which play a central role in preventing glaucoma. And so, just like hyaluronic acid, we need the nutrients that help support the body's ability to make its own collagen. These nutrients include vitamin C (more on that in chapter 9), copper (from chapter 1), lysine, and proline.

Both lysine and proline are amino acids—the building block of proteins. And collagen is protein, the most abundant protein in the human body, accounting for a quarter to half of all the protein throughout our body! Proline not only is needed for collagen but also for an elastic support protein called elastin that helps support the retina and blood vessels in the back of the eye. While the body can make its own proline from other amino acids, a good diet can help. Top sources for proline include fish, meats, and dairy products, as well as pistachios, hazelnuts, pecans, brown rice, and corn.

Lysine—also needed to make collagen—is an essential amino acid. The body cannot make its own lysine, and so we need it from dietary sources, for the most part the same ones high in proline. You may remember that in *Jurassic Park*, the dinosaurs were genetically engineered to have a lysine deficiency and would die within twelve hours if they did not receive lysine in their diets. It was a safety mechanism in case the dinosaurs escaped. Fortunately for us, we get plenty of lysine in our diets. Flounder, shrimp, steak, pistachios, cheese, and eggs are among the top sources. Other wonderful dietary choices include kidney beans, lima beans, black-eyed peas, corn, spinach, broccoli, mushrooms, and pecans.

Finally, is there a way to relax the drainage site of the eye? We talked about hormonal balance with diabetes and vascular health. Genistein is a bioflavonoid that has a strong estrogen hormone activity, which helps protect against osteoporosis and raises the level of the good cholesterol HDL (which helps with diabetes and macular conditions, as we learned in our discussion on boron in chapter 7). Genistein, most abundant in soybeans, may help relax the drainage site.

THE ELEMENTS OF A TWO-EDGED SWORD

We previously learned about "good" metals and metals that cause oxidation. Sometimes the same metal can be both beneficial and harmful.

Magnesium. We learned about the element magnesium in the chapter on diabetes, and magnesium is essential in maintaining vitamin B1 levels, and so by extension it is believed to be essential for protecting against glaucoma. However, a recent study has shown that higher magnesium levels increase the risk of glaucoma by 125 percent. The take-home message is that you need magnesium but must be careful not to have too much.

Selenium. Selenium, a non-metal element we learned about in chapter 1, is essential in its antioxidant roles but itself is an oxidant. And remember that it doubled the risk of developing glaucoma when higher amounts were taken daily. As we've been hearing about repeatedly, often natural sources give you that balanced approach. Garlic, for example, is high in selenium but promoted for good cardiovascular health, through its effects on blood pressure, cholesterols, and inflammation, all of which are a wonderful relief for the eye. Much of its effects are mediated by a compound within garlic called allicin, which gives garlic that smell and protects it against pests in the field that want a good vegetable meal. With garlic, you get much more than just selenium, and although it's high in selenium, it's not too high, so you won't go over on the selenium.

Vanadium. The metal element vanadium (chapter 7) may perhaps decrease pressure in the eye by turning down the bathtub faucet (although there is very limited data to support this), and so it has been widely promoted for glaucoma. However, vanadium is an oxidant and you don't want too much—you'll get all the vanadium you need through a healthy diet.

• • •

Finally, while most of what we focused on were the main rats in glaucoma, there are other important "rats" that can be nibbling on your optic nerve. Don't forget about decreasing oxidative stress (chapter 1) using nutrients such as glutathione; controlling inflammation (chapter 2) using nutrients such as bioflavonoids that target both the oxidation and inflammation; and, optimizing blood flow with nutrients such as arginine (chapter 3).

SUMMARY 8: GLAUCOMA

Glaucoma is a neurologic disorder of the nerve that connects the eye to the brain, characterized by loss of nerve fibers within this nerve.

Often patients are oblivious to glaucoma in its early stages and only notice visual problems when it is far advanced.

Clinical examination helps identify whether or not nerve fibers are lost and can identify these changes in the early stages of glaucoma.

Glaucoma often progresses slowly, and over time side vision is lost.

High pressure is not glaucoma; rather, it's a serious risk factor (one of several) for glaucoma.

The trabecular meshwork is a complex filter in the eye that helps regulate pressure.

If glaucoma is detected early enough, it is possible to slow the progress of the disease medically and nutritionally.

Important nutrients from chapter 8:

- Vitamin B1—essential in the pathway that makes the body's energy packets and protects neural cells from injury.
- Choline—an essential amine that forms neurotransmitters (signaling molecules).
- *Coleus forskohlii*—a mint that increases production of an important signaling molecule—called cAMP—inside cells.
- Proline—an amino acid that is needed for collagen formation.
- Lysine—an amino acid that is also needed for collagen formation.
- Magnesium—an element that is essential in maintaining vitamin B1 levels.
- Selenium—an element that in high amounts can increase the risk of glaucoma.
- Vanadium—a metal that may decrease eye pressure.
- Allicin—a compound within garlic that promotes good health.

CHAPTER 9

CATARACTS: FOGGY VISION

Papa Bear George Halas—extraordinary football player, coach, and founder of the Chicago Bears—once said, "If you live long enough, lots of nice things happen." The Yiddish saying goes, "If you live long enough, you'll see everything." When it comes to your eyes, though, if you live long enough, you'll see less and less as you gradually develop a cataract—something that is bound to happen to everyone who lives long enough. In the United States, cataracts affect 44 percent of all adults over the age of 55. The World Health Organization (WHO) estimates that cataracts are responsible for half of all blindness around the world. In less developed parts of the world, there may be little or no access to cataract surgery. Fortunately, in the United States where the surgery is widely available, cataracts are relatively easy to treat.

Cataracts primarily affect people over the age of fifty-five. A person with cataracts slowly loses vision thanks to a clouding of the lens that normally focuses light to the retina.

The lens inside the eye looks and acts like a camera lens, but it is actually a transparent watery bag of well-aligned proteins. The bag is a very thin, clear, lentil-bean–shaped sack inside of which is a crystal-like substance composed of about two-thirds water and one-third protein. The proteins are precisely arranged within long thin clear fiber cells that are organized in layers like the rings of an onion.

However, over time, as new layers of fiber cells compress old fiber cells, the clarity of the lens starts to decrease. In addition, as the lens proteins degrade and crosslink and lose alignment, they don't allow light to pass through clearly. The lens loses its clarity, often in a gradual process.

People with cloudy lenses—cataracts—have difficulty seeing clearly. Their vision is like looking through a foggy window or a steamy shower door. Just as initially when you turn on the shower's hot water there isn't much fogginess on the bathroom mirror, over time the fogginess gets worse and worse. With cataracts this is often a slow progression over years. Many times, the cloudiness develops a yellow hue, causing people to have trouble distinguishing colors and the world to look like those old yellow-brown "sepia" photographs.

Some people will complain of glare when looking at bright lights, such as lamppost lights at night or oncoming headlights. When these bright lights hit the lens with its misarranged proteins and compressed lens fibers, light does not pass through properly and a significant portion of the light starts to scatter. It scatters in all sorts of directions inside the eye to various parts of the retina. As the light does not land in the proper place in the retina to form the correct image of the outside world, it instead triggers a splattering of cells throughout the retina, which perceive the stimulus as glare.

TYPES AND CAUSES OF CATARACTS

There are many types of cataracts, depending on how the lens is affected and what part of the lens is affected. In some cases, just the back of the lens becomes cloudy, while others involve the whole lens. Sometimes the cataract is very mild and barely affects vision, while other times the cataract is quite extensive and blocks out all vision. In these cases, the cataract becomes a dark brown color or a dense white color—in fact, that is where the word cataract comes from: the Latin word for waterfall, as the dense white cataracts look like white waterfalls.

While age is the most common cause of cataracts, there are many other causes. An injury to the eye can result in the lens fibers and proteins becoming physically misaligned. An inflammatory condition that affects the eye can do the same to the fibers and proteins, though the changes happen on a much more molecular rather than physical level. Genetic syndromes can result in cataracts in infants and children. Even some medications, such as steroids, can cause cataracts. In diabetes, excess sugars cause a certain type of sugar-alcohol—called sorbitol—to form throughout the body, and this sugar-alcohol starts to accumulate within the lens and get trapped there, pulling in excess fluid with it and causing oxidative damage and degeneration of the lens proteins, resulting in earlier onset cataracts.

PREVENTING CATARACTS

The treatment of cataracts often focuses on surgery—removing the cataract lens and replacing it with a clear plastic lens. In World War II, British air force eye surgeon Sir Harold Ridley noted that when the acrylic windows of fighter planes shattered, bits and pieces of the acrylic would sometimes lodge within the eyes of aircraft pilots and ball turret gunners—but the body didn't reject these pieces of acrylic. He then proposed molding a piece of acrylic into the shape of an eye lens and using that to replace a cataract. It worked! And we've been doing it ever since, though techniques have been much more refined.

But what about preventing cataracts before they get to the point where vision is impaired? Nutrition can't reverse the changes once they occur, but as with all age-related vision conditions, the onset of cataracts can be delayed by eating a nutrient-rich diet throughout your life. The eye naturally bathes the lens in fluids that contain the highest nutrient concentration of anywhere in our bodies—it does so to protect the lens and prevent age-related cataract changes. We can help our body by ensuring the nutrients in the fluids are available for our eye to use by eating foods that contain them.

Vitamin C

There are plenty of studies that show that taking vitamins does not prevent or slow down the formation of cataracts. So shouldn't we just end here? Well, remember in chapter 1, we reviewed a study of almost twenty-five thousand women, which showed that those who took vitamin C had a higher incidence of cataracts than those who didn't take the extra dose of vitamin C. The excess vitamin C—without an appropriate balance of antioxidants—resulted in oxidation of the vitamin C into a chemical called dehydroascorbate that caused sugars to attach to proteins within the lens, damaging the lens proteins in a similar way to how diabetes causes cataracts.

You may say that was only one study—but it wasn't: The finding has been replicated. An even larger study of more than thirty-one thousand men showed the same thing—the risk of cataracts nearly doubled in older men taking only vitamin C. And the study showed an increased risk of cataracts in those who took only vitamin E—also recall from chapter 1 that vitamin E in excess and not balanced with other nutrients can act as an oxidant and block other antioxidants. And because the body preferentially distributes nutrients to the fluid around the lens to bathe the lens in these nutrients—the risks get magnified with the lens.

So the answer is that vitamins by themselves are not the answer. You need a balanced approach with multiple nutrients. Getting your nutrients through whole natural foods often gives you the extra nutrients needed for that balanced approach.

The evidence from dozens of clinical trials—and animal model studies—suggests that vitamin C is beneficial in conjunction with other nutrients in protecting the lens from damage that leads to cataract formation. No discussion of vitamin C would be complete without at least mentioning that vitamin C has been studied for other eye conditions, particularly in preventing or treating macular degeneration. The vast majority of the studies, however, show no evidence to suggest that vitamin C helps with macular degeneration.

Again, we need to take that evidence with a grain of salt—or better yet, we should take it with other nutrients. Vitamin C is a powerful antioxidant that can protect the cells throughout the eye from oxidative damage; can protect the cells in the retina from light damage by helping form melanin pigment that absorbs excess light that could damage the retina; and helps build collagen to strengthen capillaries, the optic nerve, and the filtration drain in the eye that we learned about during our discussion on glaucoma (chapter 8).

So while the US Institute of Medicine's recommended dietary allowance (RDA) of vitamin C is just under 100 mg per day with an upper limit of intake not to exceed 2,000 mg per day, should we then adhere to the vitamin C dosing parameters from a glaucoma-prevention study from the 1960s that showed that doses of vitamin C in the range of 25,000 to 50,000 mg per day lowered eye pressure? Clearly the vast array of scientific evidence suggests a balanced approach with moderation.

Vitamin A and Carotenoids

And this same type of guidance can be gleaned from studies on other nutrients, such as vitamin A and carotenoids. We've learned quite a lot about these nutrients in previous chapters, and there are indeed quite a few studies on their role in cataracts. One study of over fifty thousand women followed over eight years showed moderate decreased risks of cataracts associated with increased dietary—not pills—intake of vitamin A (primarily from animal sources and fortified foods) and carotenoids (primarily from fruits and vegetables).

An interesting study from 1991 drives home the recommendation for nutrients from natural whole foods, showing a large decrease in cataract development in people who regularly drank more than two cups of bioflavonoid-rich tea per day.

Some B-Complex Vitamins

The jury is still out on the intake of B-complex vitamins—notably B1, B2, B3, and B6—in prevention of cataracts. And the same goes for these vitamins in the prevention of macular degeneration. There is some evidence to suggest a benefit, and other evidence to suggest the contrary. Overall, though, as we delve into the mechanisms of action of these vitamins, we'll see that we need them, and we should seek to obtain a well-balanced level of them in our diets. We previously learned about the original "vital-amine"—vitamin B1—in chapter 8 on glaucoma. We also learned a lot about folate—also known as vitamin B9—in chapter 4 on our genes. Let's learn a bit about the others.

Out of the eight total B-complex vitamins, there's very little data on vitamin B5 (pantothenic acid) and the human lens. Similarly there's not much on vitamin B7 (biotin). B7 is also known as vitamin H—the "H" for the German words for hair and skin—because it helps promote healthy hair, skin, and nails. It also helps regulate and process sugars and aids proper metabolism within our cells. Vitamin B5 helps the body create energy and make lipids—specialized fats—that are essential for neural tissue in the retina and optic nerve, and plays a role—among many roles—in the production of hormones and neural signaling molecules. However, high amounts of vitamin B5 can increase the risk of bleeding.

Vitamin B2—also known as riboflavin—has many functions, including assisting enzymes in forming packets of energy within cells, supporting the production of building blocks of proteins, and sustaining the production of neural signaling molecules. It promotes antioxidant enzymes and acts with folate as an indirect antioxidant by reducing the toxin homocysteine (discussed in chapter

4). It is essential for the formation of the enzyme that creates the powerful antioxidant glutathione (that we learned about in chapter 1). It is in this role with glutathione that vitamin B2 has been believed for nearly a century to prevent cataracts.

However, vitamin B2 is a "cellular photosensitizer"—it absorbs light and becomes energetically excited, changing its shape to pull in electrons and create oxidants. So this antioxidant can suddenly turn into an oxidant, causing for example the clear lens in the eye to gradually turn brown and develop cataracts over time. There's evidence that it may exacerbate macular degeneration—with all the light that hits the retina—through this "photosensitization" resulting in excess oxidation in the retina. The antioxidant properties of vitamin C and alpha-lipoic acid can mitigate the light-toxicity effects of vitamin B2. A similar message keeps repeating: not too much, not too little—and balanced with other nutrients. Good food sources for vitamin B2 include eggs, dairy products, mushrooms, spinach, chickpeas, squash, pecans, cashews, walnuts, salmon, and flounder.

Vitamin B3 is also known as niacin—or nicotinic acid—because it was first isolated during a chemical process involving nicotine in tobacco. It is vital for energy production and is required for the function of several dozen enzymes. It is believed to lower cholesterol, protect neural cells from injury—particularly in the retina and optic nerve, which are affected in retinal conditions and glaucoma—and may even decrease blood sugars in diabetes.

Remember Jane from chapter 1, who developed blurred vision from swelling in her retina from taking a "stress-relief" formulation of B-complex vitamins, which included too much vitamin B3? Vitamin B3 can also cause a transient warm, red, itchy flush in the skin, and when too much is taken it can cause dry eye, eyelid swelling, discoloration of the eyelids, loss of eyelashes, loss of eyebrows, and bulging out of the eye. Natural sources of B3 include peanuts, sunflower seeds, haddock, tuna, salmon, chicken, and steak. Good vegetable choices include asparagus, artichoke, corn, red peppers, lima beans, peas, lentils, baked potatoes, and mushrooms.

Vitamin B6 is actually a family of vitamins called pyridoxine, pyridoxal, and pyridoxamine. This family assists dozens of enzymes within the body, helps produce energy packets within cells, and is required for the creation of neural signaling molecules. Along with zinc, vitamin B6 can convert the toxic homocysteine into the powerhouse antioxidant glutathione. Vitamin B6 can boost the immune defense system and facilitate the production of red blood cells that carry vital oxygen throughout the body. And just like vitamin B3, it can protect neural cells in the retina and optic nerve from injury.

Jane from chapter 1 also took excess B6 that caused headaches. Too much of the vitamin B6 family can also cause nerve disturbances in the arms and legs, including shooting pains, numbness, and difficulties with balance. Abdominal pains, upset stomach, and nausea are among the gastrointestinal side effects.

"Enough is enough," recently declared a team of researchers from the Johns Hopkins Medical Institutions in one of our major medical journals. "Stop wasting money on vitamin and mineral supplements." While I don't necessarily advocate giving up on nutrient supplements, I certainly encourage a balanced approach—and highly recommend that you don't overdo any one nutrient. As I've said over and over, natural sources are often the best way to go.

Natural balanced sources for vitamin B6 include walnuts, pistachios, and chestnuts. Salmon, cod, chicken, and steak as well as bananas, sweet potatoes, chili peppers, brussels sprouts, and spinach also provide healthy amounts of this nutrient, along with a whole range of other nutrients.

Vitamin D: No Laughing Matter

Vitamin D is known for its ability to decrease the winter seasonal "blues." The body needs sunlight to produce its own vitamin D, so with decreased sunlight exposure during winter, vitamin D levels in the body decrease. And that's what happened to Raymond. He spent all day indoors on the job, and when he left for work during the winter, it was already dark. His friend recommended some vitamin D and, since he was over sixty, he and his wife also started taking calcium to keep their bones strong. Raymond's mood improved, and he got rid of those nasty blues. He was doing quite well, but after some years, he slowly noted that his vision started to decrease and his eyes were always irritated. He thought that it must be cataracts developing, as that's what happens to those his age. The irritation just kept getting worse, and when I saw him for the first time and examined his eyes, there was a thin band of white calcium deposits that I could see layered on top of his corneas, drying out his corneas, irritating his eyes, and causing his vision to become hazy. It wasn't cataracts—it was too much vitamin D and calcium. Over years, it caused excess calcium to build up on the surface of Raymond's eyes, in a process called "band keratopathy." With some special eyedrops and a change from vitamin D and calcium pills to balanced natural sources, the calcium buildup went away, his vision cleared, and the irritation disappeared.

It is known that vitamin D deficiency causes depression, weakness, and sleepiness. Vitamin D also supports the immune defense system—protecting against the common cold—and is believed to decrease high blood pressure. Low levels of vitamin D have been associated with cardiovascular disease, certain types of cancer, and neurodegenerative processes such as Alzheimer's disease. However, there is mounting evidence that vitamin D does little for bone health—that is, without appropriate calcium intake. With calcium, vitamin D does indeed help our bones.

Vitamin D is actually not a true vitamin—it is a steroid hormone, known as calciferol. And it actually does not do anything. Yes, I did say that correctly: Vitamin D cannot perform any actions whatsoever. It gets converted through a series of reactions to a specialized molecule—called 25-hydroxyvitamin D2—which is able to go inside the nucleus of cells and turn on genes within the cells—and it can actually turn on some fifty different genes within our cells. Remember from chapter 4 that those are not the genes that change our traits—think eye color or hair color—but the genes that affect day-to-day functioning of our cells.

The existing research does not give us a clear indication of vitamin D's benefits for preventing cataracts or macular degeneration. These lettered vitamins are all needed for the balanced approach. Go for your vitamin D-rich foods, such as dairy and fish, particularly herring, flounder, and salmon. But be sure to add fruits and vegetables that will give you the B-complex vitamins and all the other nutrients the body needs for its complex and intricate molecular, cellular, and physiological activities.

SUMMARY 9: CATARACTS

A cataract is a clouding of the lens inside the eye that focuses light from the front of the eye to the back of the eye.

There are many types of cataracts, depending on how the lens is affected and what part of the lens is affected.

While age is the most common cause of cataracts, there are many other causes, including injury, inflammation, genetic syndromes, medications, and diabetes.

To protect the lens, it is naturally bathed in fluids that contain the highest nutrient concentration of anywhere in our bodies. We can help our bodies protect the lens with good nutrition.

Important nutrients from chapter 9:

- Vitamin C—a powerful antioxidant that protects the lens.

- Vitamin B2—assists in forming energy packets and promotes antioxidant enzymes but also acts as a photosensitizer to create electrons.

- Vitamin B3—assists with energy production and protects neural cells from injury.

- Vitamin B6—assists with many enzymes including those involved in energy production.

- Vitamin D—actually a steroid hormone that turns on genes within our cells.

CHAPTER 10

DRY EYE: NO MORE TEARS

Wendy was a high-powered executive who spent hours on the computer every day. She complained that at the end of the day, her eyes were red and tired and felt like there was grit in them. They teared all the time. She went to one doctor, who told her that she had dry eye and that she needed to use artificial tears. That made little sense to Wendy. Her eyes were tearing, not dry. So she didn't do anything, and by the time she came to my office (she thought there was something wrong with the back of her eye, so she came to me, a retina specialist), her condition was severe and she was worn out. I explained to her that her eyes really were dry, partly because of spending all that time reading and using the computer—the eye forgets to blink and slowly over time, it dries out. We did add some artificial tears, encouraged her to take short breaks to blink her eyes, and instituted some dietary change, including adding fish to her diet along with more vegetables, particularly sweet potatoes, carrots, kale, and collard greens. After a month, Wendy's symptoms resolved and she couldn't thank me enough.

In a world where most people look at computer screens and smartphones for hours every day, one in seven Americans of all ages has a medical condition called dry eye. In fact, dry eye is the most common vision-related disorder.

WHAT IS DRY EYE?

Dry eye is a disorder of the surface of the eye in which there is an imbalance in the ocular tears that lubricate the eye. The result is a dryness of the surface of the eye, notably on the surface of the cornea, the clear window of the eye that lets in light.

Since the cornea is the most sensitive part of the body (with more nerve endings per square millimeter than anywhere else in the body), it is exquisitely sensitive to even the smallest irritation, including dryness. And it needs to be so sensitive, so that it can trigger your windshield wipers—your eyelids—to clean any debris off the window: the cornea. Symptoms of dry eye include irritation of the eye, and a sensation of sand or grit in the eye—the irritation may be mild or may be disabling. Often the eye is red, at least a bit red, but it can be very red as well. Over time, vision may start to blur—it's as if you're looking through a dirty window . . . smudges, blurring, haze, and downright cloudiness. The blurred vision may be very mild or may be devastating. Other symptoms include burning and itching. There may be discharge from the eye (stuff coming out of the eye).

Often the dry eye waters. Yes, the eye is dry, but yet it waters, as the eye tries to open up the floodgates—but it is not a balanced approach. It is literally like pouring a gallon of water on top of a flower garden on a gently sloping hill . . . if the flower garden is bone dry, all of the water is going to slide all the way down the slope and the flower garden doesn't get watered.

Dry eye is diagnosed when someone comes to the office complaining of these symptoms, and the doctor looks at the cornea. The doctor can detect dryness in the cornea with a specialized eye-examining microscope (called a slit lamp biomicroscope). Sometimes, eyedrops are placed in the eye to see if the dryness has caused damage to cells on the surface of the eye (this damage is often temporary, as the cells on the surface of the cornea completely replace themselves every seven to ten days). Sometimes the eye's ability to produce tears is measured.

CAUSES OF DRY EYE

Caused by a wide variety of conditions, from menopause to long hours spent in front of a computer screen, dry eyes occur when your eyes simply don't have enough moisture. If you've ever walked into a sharp gale of wind that simply took the moisture in your eyes away, then you know the uncomfortable sting of dry eye. You may also experience dry eye every day, in the form of "tired eyes" when reading or using the computer.

Dry eye is about more than just tears, though to understand the mechanisms of dry eye you need to focus on what is happening to those tears. Mechanisms include: (1) increased tear evaporation, which for example occurs in low-humidity environments; (2) decreased tear production, which can occur when the tear glands don't produce enough tears; or, (3) unstable tear film, meaning that the actual tear film, or the thin layer of tears that coats the surface of the eye, starts to break apart leaving dry gaps. This instability may occur during contact lens wear or from inflammation of the eyelids (a disorder called blepharitis).

Dry eye happens to most people after fifty, though with the growing reliance on and prevalence of screen time, the condition has become relatively ubiquitous across all age groups. A major cause of dry eye is not blinking often enough, which is what happens when you concentrate your vision on a screen or read.

The most common cause of dry eye is aging, as we produce less tears as we age, and the quality of the tears that we produce decreases as we age. Dry eye is more common in women, as a result of hormonal changes, and can be particularly bad after menopause. Environmental factors can also lead to dry eye: Hot, dry, and windy conditions outdoors, and the decreased humidity associated with air-conditioning or heating indoors. Chemical vapors and smoke can exacerbate dry eye. Irritants don't have to be in the air; alcohol and caffeine are ingested and delivered through the bloodstream. There are many medications—prescription and over-the-counter—that can cause dry eye, including over-the-counter allergy medications (antihistamines), common antidepressants, and some types of blood pressure pills. There are also many diseases with an inflammatory component that may contribute to dry eye, including lupus, rheumatoid arthritis, and Sjögren's syndrome. We spoke about diabetes in chapter 7.

Treatment for dry eye is focused on replenishing the tears, preventing or minimizing the loss of tears, and adding additional protection to the ocular surface. Artificial teardrops—that you buy in an over-the-counter bottle or small tubes—are often a balanced salt solution and are the most common way to treat dry eye. But human tears are much more than a balanced salt solution.

BEYOND CROCODILE TEARS

What are tears? Scientists believe that the tears we produce to express our emotions are unique to humans. Have you seen your pet dog or cat tear up? They can produce tears, but they serve a lubricating function and do not express emotion. Other animals "cry" but without tears. Often, it's the young offspring of the animals that cry, usually just verbal expressions of sorrow. Recently, a baby elephant was observed to cry with tears after his mother savagely cast him out. But was that crying due to an emotional response or from physical injuries as he was disowned? What about the crocodile tears of sorrow that drip down their scaly faces when a crocodile eats a human? Those liquid tears have been observed for hundreds of years. But is a crocodile sad when it eats a human? Does it feel remorse? Or is it faking remorse? Researchers have indeed observed crocodiles tearing up when eating, sometimes quite extensively. There may be a tearing reflex that occurs when the crocodiles eat, or perhaps it is simply the need for a crocodile to lubricate its eyes when it is out of the water such as when munching on a meal.

So there are three different types of tears. In addition to the tears of emotion—unique to humans—there are the lubricating tears, which come in two types: those that are constantly produced to lubricate the eyes (called basal tears) and those that are produced in response to an irritant to the eye (called reflex tears). Dry eye is caused by a problem with the lubricating tears.

So let's get down to the science of tears—what you ask, a *science* of tears—yes, tears are much more than just salty water.

Tears not only deliver nutrients to the eye's surface; they also remove excess debris and waste from the surface and create an additional layer of protection on the surface of the eye—called the tear film—which also serves to smooth out the surface of the cornea so that the light that enters the eye is a smoothly focused image. It's like having a special liquid coating on your glasses or on your camera lens that improves the quality of the image that goes through the lens.

With every blink you take, your eyelids squeeze a little microscopic bit of oil out of rows of microscopic oil glands within your eyelids located right next to where your lashes come out of your lids. This oil mixes with the electrolyte (salt) balanced solution that the tear gland—located underneath the outer edge of the upper eyelid—produces. The oils give the tears some thickness and keep them more viscous in order to prevent evaporation. Tears contain antibodies and proteins to fight off infections—in fact, there are dozens of different types of proteins mixed into tears. Some promote the growth of surface cells while others serve to signal important biochemical processes.

Tears are even full of nutrients and vitamins. You could collect a bit of a stash of vitamin C just by crying . . . and some vitamin A and other nutrients too. These nutrient-rich tears nourish the surface cells of the eye. Remember how we learned about the amazingly sophisticated front of the eye, with its own set of living stem cells that constantly regenerate to replenish and fully replace the entire surface of the cornea every week or so. Well, tears are essential to properly nourishing these cells.

SOME NUTRIENTS TO INCLUDE IN THE MIX

Eating specific foods, combined with small lifestyle choices (like taking hourly breaks from your computer screen or making sure to blink your eyes on a timed schedule when reading) can help alleviate the symptoms of dry eye substantially, just as they did for Wendy. Often these changes will work quickly, while it may take much longer in more severe cases.

It has been known since antiquity that vitamin A deficiency causes a severe type of dry eye called xerophthalmia, where the surface of the eye becomes so dry and thick that infections can easily develop and the cornea can thin out and develop craters in its surface that ultimately open into the eye—a serious vision-threatening condition called an ulcer. It is a blinding condition treated easily with vitamin A. While xerophthalmia is exceedingly uncommon in the United States, it reinforces the importance of vitamin A in our diets, and studies have shown that vitamin A can improve the stability of the tears and effectively treat dry eye. It can also promote a healthy immune system—needed for protection of the surface of the eye—by supporting the function of white blood cells. Vitamin A has also been demonstrated to promote the regeneration of healthy cells on the surface of the eye. Go for your squash, pumpkin, asparagus, sweet peppers, and cantaloupe in addition to other top sources of vitamin A we've previously mentioned.

As a powerful antioxidant, vitamin C is essential for the surface of the eye. Keeping the cells healthy so they can create the right kind of lubricating tears and keep the surface clear and functioning properly is a top priority for proper vision. Vitamin C is required for the production of mucins—complexes of proteins bound with sugars—that allow the tear film—that thin layer of tears on the surface of the eye—to adhere gently to the surface and coat the surface.

Vitamin C has many roles. We've talked about its antioxidant properties in chapter 1, about its collagen-building activities in chapter 8 on glaucoma, and about its help in protecting against cataracts in chapter 9. In addition, it is believed to decrease the risk of heart disease and heart attacks. It may strengthen capillaries and reduce cholesterol levels. There's even some suggestion that it may decrease the risk of certain types of cancer, including breast cancer. In the back of the eye, vitamin C helps form a protein building block—amino acid—called tyrosine, which is a precursor to pigment granules called melanin that are found behind the retina and help absorb light to protect against light toxicity.

Humans are among the few living creatures who can't make their own vitamin C. So go for kiwis, strawberries, oranges, and papayas. Take in those brussels sprouts, broccoli, chile peppers, red peppers, and spinach.

A TALE OF BALANCE

In chapter 6, we learned about the importance of omega-3 oils in many eye conditions, including retinitis pigmentosa. We also found out about its benefits in dry eye, with research studies demonstrating its ability to decrease the risk of dry eye. More important, we were introduced to the concept that omega-3 oils helped block the harmful effects of omega-6 oils. These harmful effects include the promotion of abnormal blood vessel growth (which is devastating in macular degeneration and in diabetic retinopathy) and excess blood clotting. More worrisome is the ability of omega-6 oils to initiate inflammation. We dedicated a whole chapter to how to prevent inflammation. And in the context of dry eye, we want to decrease inflammation on the surface of the eye, as inflammation is one of the causative agents or exacerbators of dry eye. We called the omega-6 oils the bad fats, found in chocolate chip cookies as well as cheese, meats, and crackers.

And now, I am about to say that omega-6 oils are good for you. Let me qualify these statements and start with an explanation. Omega-6 oils are secreted by the oil glands in the eyelids, and they are part of the important oils that prevent evaporation of the lubricating tears. As such, they are essential for a healthy eye surface. But what turns out to be the most important message about omega-6 oils is that they must be balanced properly with omega-3 oils. Some of these seemingly harmful effects—inflammation, blood clotting, and new blood vessel growth—can actually be beneficial when they are in moderation, in controlled situations. A bit of inflammation may be needed to prevent infections; a bit of blood clotting can help prevent bleeding; a bit of new blood vessel growth may be helpful in certain situations. The balance between omega-6 oils and omega-3 oils can achieve this controlled moderation. In fact, omega-6 oils can serve as precursors to some omega-3 oils, such as one called eicosapenaenoic acid—or EPA for short—when the body needs them.

However, our diets are often filled with much more omega-6 oils than omega-3 oils. In fact, most people in the United States consume about ten to twenty times more omega-6 than omega-3 oils. An ideal balance for most people is somewhere between an equal one-to-one balance and a three-to-one balance with three times the amount of omega-6 oils as compared to omega-3 oils. That's why eating fewer chocolate chip cookies and increasing consumption of salmon (for example) can help achieve a balance that studies show can decrease the risk of dry eye.

• • •

As you read Part III of the book, I encourage you to think beyond the confines of the specific nutrients listed in each chapter. Preventing and treating dry eye involves much more than the vitamin A, vitamin C, and omega oils we just discussed. It involves the mix of dozens of nutrients that help protect against the many mechanisms of disease that we've been learning about throughout the book. So open up your palate and let's get to eating the healthy stuff!

As the brilliant ancient Greek physician Hippocrates supposedly said over two centuries ago, "Let food be thy medicine. . . ." And so true that is! However, despite the wide circulation of this quote, Hippocrates never said it. Which brings me to an important point: There is so much misinformation out there that it is essential to use common sense and make sure you don't overdo it with nutrients— as I've mentioned repeatedly, the best approach often is the natural whole foods approach, rather than supplements and pills. I've tried to be as careful as I can with all the data I've presented, by going through thousands of pages of medical literature over many years. And for something as personal and specific as your own health and your own body, it's always best to ask your doctor.

SUMMARY 10: DRY EYE

The most common vision-related disorder is dry eye, an ailment of the surface of the eye, in which there is an imbalance in the ocular tears that lubricate the eye.

Mechanisms of dry eye include increased tear evaporation, decreased tear production, or unstable tear film.

Tears are more than just salty water: they contain balanced electrolytes, oils, proteins, antibodies, and nutrients.

Treatment for dry eye is focused on replenishing the tears, preventing or minimizing the loss of tears, and adding additional protection to the ocular surface.

Important nutrients from chapter 10:

- Vitamin C—required for the production of an essential component of tears.

- Omega-3 oils—must be balanced with omega-6 oils to protect the eye and prevent inflammation.

- Omega-6 oils—secreted by the eyelids as an essential component for a healthy eye surface.

- Vitamin A—stabilizes tears and supports the healthy immune function of the surface of the eye.

PART III:

EATING FOR HEALING

CHAPTER 11

A VISIONARY PALATE

In this chapter, I will provide you with a list of foods that help promote eye health. This list will form a sample menu, from which you can select your diet. Within this list, there are a quite few "all-star" foods that can be particularly potent in providing you with beneficial nutrients. Keep in mind, though, that this healthy vision menu is not meant to be an exhaustive list, but rather to highlight specifics and provide you with a sample guide on how to achieve the best balance of the nutrients that our eyes need the most. Everything on the list is healthful and restorative.

I've grouped the foods into the following ten categories: vegetables, fruits, nuts, beans, fish/meat/eggs, grains, flavorings and spices, sweeteners, oils, and drinks.

As you go through this list, keep in mind that the processing or cooking of foods may degrade food or add oxidation. Let's take carotenoids, for example. Carotenoids in carrots can be degraded by oxidation, through pathways that involve heat (from cooking), exposure to oxygen (from blending or pureeing), exposure to light (also from blending or pureeing), or acids or metals or other oxidants (from mixing with other foods). Similarly, slicing fruits high in vitamin C often exposes them to light and oxygen, which starts the breakdown process of vitamin C. Eat them soon after slicing, if you're going to slice them at all. Other foods, such as tomatoes, release their nutrients when cooked, and so cooking them is better. Often, the saying is: "Keep them raw," but I believe that the easiest approach is simply to take in a mix: raw and cooked. If cooked, lightly cooking or steaming is often gentler to the enzymes and nutrients in the veggies than boiling or microwaving. As always, avoid overly processed foods.

FRUITS AND VEGETABLES: HOW MANY SERVINGS?

Let's take a small detour before we begin the list to talk about fruits and vegetables. The US Centers for Disease Control and Prevention (CDC) has stated that "almost everyone needs to eat more fruits and vegetables." That sounds like an exaggeration. Everyone? Really? But let's look at how much fruits and veggies we eat. Yesterday, for example, did you have veggies with both lunch and dinner? How many servings of veggies did you have? What about fruits? How many did you have? Many of us fall short of the amount we really need.

You may have heard the phrase "strive for five," referring to 5 servings of fruit and 5 servings of vegetables per day. That is a reasonable goal. The CDC has issued guidelines recommending that we increase our intake: up to 3 cups of fruit and up to 4 cups of vegetables per day depending on your age, sex, and level of daily physical activity. But even that may not be enough. So how do you know how much you need to get? Is it 5 servings? Is it 3 cups? What's the difference? What should you do? There are all sorts of different types of veggies and fruits. Which ones should you eat and how often? And how do you keep track of all that? It just can be dizzying.

VEGETABLES

So let's simplify it. Let's start with veggies. The healthy vision menu calls for veggies at lunch, dinner, and snack. Go for a salad as one of your full meals each day: either lunch or dinner. A medium to large salad can give you 3 or more servings of veggies, and a small to medium salad can give you at least 2 servings of veggies. If lunch was a salad, then dinner should include veggies, either as two side dishes or as a part of the dinner entree with a veggie side dish. If dinner was a salad, then lunch should include veggies on the side or as part of the entree. To round it out, you'll want to include in your day some crisp raw veggie snacks—which we'll talk about in this chapter.

As you see, you're giving yourself veggies three times during the day (lunch, dinner, and snack), and the veggies are mostly uncooked: in salads and snacks.

So what veggies are we talking about? I've divided the veggies into several categories: the leafy veggies, the everyday salad and cooking veggies, the side-dish veggies, the topping veggies, and the munchies. Feel free to mix things up as you like. Keep your own list and add your favorite veggies to your list.

Leafy Veggies

When you think of leafy veggies, you think of the many varieties of lettuce. Yes, those are going to be the essentials of a salad, but the leafy all-stars to include are spinach, kale, parsley, and red cabbage. Please don't drown your salad in dressing, but a bit of a healthy oil—such as olive oil—is critical to help your body absorb the "fat-soluble" vitamins such as A, E, D, and K and help them get from your gut into your bloodstream.

Spinach. It conjures up images of Popeye and reminders of its high iron content. Yes, it has a nice dose of iron: 4 mg per 4-ounce serving. More than that, it is loaded with vitamin A—11,000 IU per serving—that supports the light-sensing cells of the retina, protects against dry eye, and boosts immune defense. It also gives you plenty of folate—220 micrograms per serving—and numerous other nutrients. A single serving has an incredible 15 mg of lutein and zeaxanthin! You don't necessarily need to have spinach every day, but certainly make it part of your diet.

If you're on a blood thinner for a heart or cardiovascular condition, your doctor may have already asked you to avoid green leafy vegetables. That is often because of the vitamin K, and spinach does have vitamin K—a hefty 570 micrograms per serving—which can interfere with some blood thinners. Taking vitamin K in the form of a pill is quite different from these natural sources of vitamin K, as the pill form may cause vitamin K to build up in the bloodstream, whereas the body can easily store or excrete excess vitamin K from the natural veggies.

Kale. Our next leafy all-star is kale. It also has quite a bit of vitamin K, and if you thought spinach was loaded with vitamin A, then you'll be amazed with the 16,000 IU of vitamin A per 4-ounce serving of kale. And kale has even more lutein and zeaxanthin than spinach: 23 mg per serving. And it has 100 mg of bioflavonoids and 9 mg of quercetin per serving—that most active bioflavonoid that may help prevent diabetes, macular degeneration, cataracts, glaucoma, eye inflammation, and other eye conditions. And it has diindolylmethane—DIM—that potent biologically active anti-inflammatory compound. It is an all-star, fresh or cooked, though avoid boiling as that may deactivate the DIM.

Red cabbage. Turning our attention from green to purple, let's talk about red cabbage. It has a couple hundred milligrams of bioflavonoids per 4-ounce serving. It's also a wonderful source of DIM, and per serving it has 6 micrograms of sulforaphane—that amazing chemical that recruits all those antioxidant enzymes within our bodies. Weird but true, Babe Ruth used to place a piece of wet cabbage under his hat during baseball games to keep cool. A better use: salads. Mix in red cabbage with your salads every once in a while—or more! As with the kale, avoid boiling, as that may decrease the available DIM and sulforaphane.

Parsley. We don't think of parsley as the star of a salad, but it certainly can supplement any salad. As such, you probably won't get a full 4-ounce serving in a single meal, but even if you get a small amount, you'll end up with quite a bit of lutein and zeaxanthin and other nutrients. Four ounces will get you 270 mg of bioflavonoids, or more. It is also loaded with 1,900 micrograms of vitamin K per serving.

Everyday Salad and Cooking Veggies

Some basic everyday veggies to include in the healthy vision menu are tomatoes, onions, corn, and peppers. Not much sounds exciting about this group, and that's why I call them the basics. You can cook them with meals—but don't overcook them—or add them to salads. They're an important component of your healthy diet.

Tomatoes. One of the most commonly eaten vegetables around the world, tomatoes are technically fruits not vegetables, as they develop from tomato flowers and contain seeds within them. They are highly versatile—good for salads, meals, soups, and sauces—think pasta sauce. A 4-ounce serving of tomato will get you 3 mg of lycopene, that red carotenoid that serves as a powerful antioxidant. It has a healthy 10 mg of glutathione to fight that war against oxidation. It's one reason Mediterranean cuisine is healthy.

Onions. Chop them, sauté them, roast them, you name it, they're a good addition to your meals. But not your eyes: chopping onions releases enzymes within the onion that create a gas that floats up through the air and irritates the surface of the eye, triggering a tearing reaction, which serves the purpose of flushing out the irritant. Onions have some bioflavonoids, consisting mostly of quercetin—about 40 mg per 4-ounce serving—much more than kale, and perhaps one of the best sources of quercetin. A single serving of onions will also give you some 200 or so micrograms of boron, which helps with hormonal balance and prevention of macular degeneration.

Corn. This vegetable traces its roots back thousands of years to the ancient indigenous Mayans and Olmecs of the Americas. Corn has a bit of everything: From carotenoids and antioxidant phytonutrients to some of the lettered vitamins to some amino acids, it's a good all-around addition, though perhaps not an all-star that shines in any one category. It makes for a good side dish, for a good topping to salads—and popping it is a healthy choice. As popcorn, it retains most of its nutrients and makes for a wonderful snack or dessert. Avoid the extra butter and salt—just some light oil is fine. Also, air pop it, and avoid the microwavable bags with extra ingredients and plasticized inner linings.

Peppers. With all the different types of peppers, let's keep our "basics" list down to three: green peppers, red peppers, and red hot pepper or chile peppers. The sweet red peppers have multiple nutrients to help your eyes. They have 8 mg of glutathione per serving, along with beta-carotene, 200 mg of vitamin C, about 4 IU of vitamin E, and nearly 4,000 IU of vitamin A per serving! Green peppers are a good all-around source of bioflavonoids and contain troxerutin, a bioflavonoid that helps with blood circulation. As with the red, the green also has vitamin C, vitamin E, and vitamin A, though not quite as much as the red. Red hot chile peppers also have vitamin A, C, and E to a similar extent as the green, but they are loaded with quercetin, about 40 mg per 4-ounce serving, in the same range as onions. So just like onions, go ahead and chop them, cook them, sauté them, roast them—get them into your diet.

Side-Dish Veggies

Some veggies just scream out "side dish" though they don't necessarily have to be relegated to that position. Having them in your side-dish rotation, though, is certainly a wise choice. These all-star side-dish veggies include sweet potatoes, squash, brussels sprouts, and asparagus.

Sweet Potatoes. We learned in chapter 5 on macular degeneration about the long lives of people living in the "Blue Zones" whose diets include copious amounts of sweet potatoes and other carotenoids. Remember that the world's oldest-ever human in documented history ate pumpkins and sweet potatoes three times per day. Sweet potatoes are loaded with vitamin A: 22,000 IU per 4-ounce serving! They are also a wonderful source of many other nutrients, including 4 mg of the antioxidant coenzyme Q10 that also helps produce energy and digest debris. So go for the baked sweet potato several times per week—or more, if you are so inclined!

Squash. With its many varieties—summer, acorn, yellow crook-neck, butternut, spaghetti, even pumpkin—squash can be used in many versatile ways as side dishes or as part of your entree, salad, soup, or even dessert. They are wonderful sources for your carotenoids: beta-carotene for those squashes whose meat is more orange and lutein and zeaxanthin for those squashes whose meat is more yellow. With a wide variety of other nutrients, they also are a wonderful source of antioxidants such as glutathione, with 10 to 15 mg per 4-ounce serving.

Brussels sprouts. These Belgian vegetables—it is believed that they originated from northern Europe—that look like small cabbages are known by many kids around the world as public-enemy number one! However, they belong near the top of your go-for-it veggie list, with a broad range of nutrients, including healthy loads of the lettered vitamins such as 100 mg of vitamin C per serving. More important, they are a wonderful source of DIM and sulforaphane, containing about 9 micrograms of sulforaphane per serving. Steam, sauté, or grill them, but avoid boiling them as that is known to deactivate the sulforaphane.

Asparagus. This succulent vegetable is known as the "food of kings" for its popularity among Roman emperors and European kings, particularly King Louis XIV of France, who wrote poetry about asparagus and created greenhouses to cultivate it year-round. With antioxidants and phytochemicals such as troxerutin, it's a good choice. A single 4-ounce serving gets you 33 mg of glutathione as well as 200 micrograms of folate.

Topping Veggies

I call this category the "topping veggies"—the garnishing veggies—as they can be added on top of salads, sandwiches, and other meals, but you can use them for many purposes. My list is fairly short—mushrooms, broccoli sprouts, and avocado—but feel free to expand your list of topping veggies with your favorites.

Mushrooms. These fungi come in thousands of varieties, including many fatally poisonous types. Of the edible types, let's focus on the common white button mushroom and the more mature version of the same species—the portobello. Back in chapter 2, we learned about how these mushrooms contain lectins that help control inflammation. They also have other nutrients, including a half milligram of vitamin B2, 4 mg of vitamin B3, and 150 IU of vitamin D per 4-ounce serving. They have metal nutrients, such as 0.4 mg of copper, 2 mg of iron, and 0.6 mg of zinc per serving. Just be careful not to have too many mushrooms because of the selenium—it has 11 micrograms per serving. And they have protein building blocks—amino acids—such as 40 mg per serving of methionine, which serves as a precursor to antioxidants and helps remove debris behind the retina.

Broccoli sprouts. While they may look like alfalfa sprouts, they have more of a bite of crispy bitterness to them. Where they excel is in their content of sulforaphane—about 300 micrograms per serving. It's best to eat them fresh and add them to your diet multiple times per week. They are an easy topping!

Avocado. Spreadable and edible, this culinary vegetable is technically a fruit, used for centuries in the Americas, dating back to the Middle Stone Age, some ten thousand years BC. Used for dips, spreads, and toppings, it is a nice "creamy" addition that's much healthier than butter and other condiments. With 32 mg of glutathione per 4-ounce serving, as well as a wide variety of the lettered vitamins including nearly 100 micrograms of folate and a healthy balance of metal nutrients, it is certainly a good choice. Avocado also has oils that help absorb the fat-soluble vitamins. Ongoing research is exploring other phytonutrients in avocados.

The Munchies

Veggies that you can snack on all day long for low-calorie nutrition—let's call those the munchies. Commonly, you see carrots and broccoli on snack trays with ranch dressing. Yes, sure, go for some ranch dressing with them—just the slightest dab though—and it will help your body absorb the fat-soluble vitamins. You don't have to limit these veggies to only munching them at snack time—you can add them to salads, or create side dishes and entrees. As with the other categories of veggies, feel free to expand your list of munchies.

Carrots. Yes, eating carrots is good for your eyes. It goes without saying. With 19,000 IU of vitamin A, a single 4-ounce serving of carrots serves up a tremendous benefit. And, as we've discussed previously, with a healthy liver, your body can control the amount of vitamin A it receives from carrots, as opposed to vitamin A pills that can overdose you. Carrots have multiple other nutrients, as well as amino acids: 100 mg each of arginine—for infection protection and blood flow—and lysine and proline—for collagen formation. And it doesn't stop there: Carrots also include coenzyme Q10, glutathione, and debris-busting phytic acid.

Broccoli. We had quite a lively discussion on broccoli back in chapter 2 on inflammation. With its abundance of bioflavonoids, quercetin, DIM, sulforaphane, and glutathione, broccoli certainly goes a long way to helping your eyes and your vision. In addition, it has higher amounts of those same amino acids that carrots have. It has 100 mg of vitamin C per serving and 10 mg of coenzyme Q10 per 4-ounce serving. Avoid the hard boil that may decrease the efficacy of the DIM and sulforaphane—go for it fresh, sautéed, steamed, or grilled.

FRUITS

As we're starting to see, a typical vegetable contains multiple nutrients that can help maintain vision. The same goes for fruits. As with vegetables, organic fruits will contain less pesticide residue than their non-organic counterparts. In either case, though, please do wash your fruits and veggies.

We'll talk about five categories: citrus fruits, berries, melons, the "everyday" fruits, and tropical or exotic fruits. Just a word of caution: diabetics must limit sugar intake and may not be able to eat as much fruit as non-diabetics. Fruits are certainly a better option than other types of sweets. Nevertheless, diabetics should consult their doctor about how much fruit they can eat per day and about replacing portions of fruit with vegetables.

Fruits make for wonderful snacks and desserts. Getting in one serving per day of each of the five categories is a good way to start. But feel free to rotate the selections around. By no means is this list meant to be exhaustive—add your own favorites to this healthy vision menu.

Citrus Fruits

Oranges, tangerines, grapefruit, and lemons. They can be eaten fresh, squeezed for juice, or incorporated into many types of dishes, notably desserts. Though they're known for their vitamin C levels, they tend to have only modest amounts of vitamin C: about 50 mg per 4-ounce serving. Their true benefit is in the variety of other nutrients they contain. They all have healthy portions of bioflavonoids—from 40 to 60 mg per 4-ounce serving. Grapefruit—from the pink to the ruby red—are wonderful sources for lycopene: about 2 mg per serving. All citrus fruits will get you nearly 10 mg or even more glutathione per serving for even more antioxidant benefit.

Berries

Strawberries, blueberries, raspberries, and blackberries. Deliciously sweet and often with a tang, there are numerous different types of berries. What most—and certainly this group of four berries—share is a load of bioflavonoids. Blueberries and blackberries contain the most, with 200 to 400 mg per 4-ounce serving, while strawberries and raspberries have a generous but comparatively small 50 mg per serving. Some are high in quercetin, such as blueberries with 6 mg per serving, while strawberries lead the group with 70 mg of vitamin C per serving. They will certainly provide a boost to the body's antioxidant capabilities and many other nutritional benefits.

Melons

Watermelon. It's a member of the cucumber and squash family and has been recently voted as the official state vegetable of Oklahoma, though scientifically it is a fruit and some classify it as a berry. Good for juicing, grilling, or just plain fresh and cold, it's an all-star of fruits. It has more antioxidant lycopene—at 5 mg per 4-ounce serving—than tomatoes. It also has a whole host of other nutrients, including 8 mg of glutathione per serving.

Cantaloupe. The orange color means it's full of beta-carotene: about 3 mg per 4-ounce serving. As with watermelon, it has numerous other nutrients and the same 8 mg of glutathione per serving. Eat it fresh or use it for desserts, sorbets, smoothies, or even a cold soup.

Everyday Fruits

Apples, pears, peaches, and bananas. These are the most common fruit staples. While they may not be all-stars in any one particular category of nutrient, they contain a modest amount of a variety of nutrients. They have about 10 to 25 mg of bioflavonoids per 4-ounce serving—with pears having the most and apples having the least. Pears and apples are high in quercetin, while peaches and apples contain troxerutin. Glutathione is present in a moderate amount in peaches, pears, and apples, as is boron—about 300 to 600 micrograms per serving. While bananas have less boron and glutathione, they lead the group with vitamin C—though it is only a small amount: 10 mg. So go for these "common" fruits—add them into your weekly or even daily rotation.

Tropical or Exotic Fruits

Kiwis, mangoes, and pomegranates. While these three fruits are not necessarily tropical or exotic, they are colorful and have unique tastes. They are nutritional all-stars. Kiwis are loaded with over 100 mg of vitamin C per 4-ounce serving. They even have a fair amount of vitamin K—nearly 50 micrograms per serving. Mangoes are moderately high in vitamin C—30 mg per serving—and folate—50 micrograms per serving. They also contain a good amount of glutathione, 6 mg per serving. Pomegranates have bioflavonoids, quite a bit of vitamin A (1,200 IU per serving), and a modest amount of vitamin C (40 mg per serving) and folate (50 micrograms per serving). They are loaded with a unique group of antioxidant chemicals called ellagitannins—also found in red raspberries—that are the subject of numerous ongoing studies on their health benefits. The seeds are edible and contain fiber and a bit of healthy oils. For desserts, juicing, or just eating fresh, these fruits are certainly good choices.

NUTS

Beloved favorite of squirrels, nuts are technically fruits that are dried and have hard shells. They are generally a good source of energy and protein. They do have fats, but because of their beneficial omega-3 oils, the oils are a good balanced source. In fact, researchers have shown that because of the oil spectrum in nuts and because they have a group of compounds called phytosterols—that block absorption of cholesterol in your gut—nuts in moderation may decrease levels of "bad" LDL cholesterol, which is a main cause of heart and blood vessel disease. So by improving your heart and blood vessels, you're doing your eyes and vision a big favor.

Almonds, Cashews, Chestnuts, Hazelnuts, Peanuts, Pecans, Pine Nuts, Pistachios, and Walnuts

While you may want to avoid or limit your intake of Brazil nuts because of their high amount of selenium, these other nuts provide a wide variety of nutrients. Overall, as a group, they provide the following metals: iron, copper, zinc, magnesium, and manganese. They provide the following amino acids: arginine, methionine, lysine, and proline. In addition, they'll get you a host of vitamins: B1, B2, B3, B6, E, and folate.

Starting with the metals, you'll be in for a good 4 to 6 mg of iron per 4-ounce serving. Chestnuts have the least of the metal nutrients, while cashews have a bit more. They'll provide you with some copper, ranging generally from 1 to 2 mg per serving—though cashews have a bit more at 2.5 mg and chestnuts a bit less at 0.5 mg per serving. Balance that copper out with zinc, at 2.5 to 4 mg per serving—though cashews (6.5 mg per serving) and pecans (5.1 mg per serving) have a bit more, and chestnuts a bit less at 1.0 mg per serving. They all have a good 140 to 220 mg of magnesium, though cashews and almonds have a bit more at 300 mg and chestnuts a bit less at 30 mg per serving. They'll all give you between 1.4 to 2.5 mg of manganese per serving, with hazelnuts giving you 7.0 mg, pecans giving you 5.1 mg, and walnuts giving you 4.4 mg.

We know that nuts shine with protein, some better than others. For arginine—the amino acid that helps with blood flow—walnuts

147

will give you a very generous 4,000 mg per serving and peanuts, 3,500 mg. On the other end, chestnuts are the least protein-rich of this group and will give you only 100 mg. The remainder of the group will give you 1,300 to 2,800 mg per serving. The same holds for methionine, the energy-boosting and debris-busting amino acid. With the exception of chestnuts, these nuts will afford you 200 to 500 mg per serving. For the collagen-forming lysine and proline, the nuts are all top choices—600 to 1,300 mg of lysine and 900 to 1,300 mg of proline—except for chestnuts which have the least amount of protein and hazelnuts and pecans, which have only a moderate amount of lysine and proline.

In terms of the lettered vitamins, they'll afford you some vitamins B1, B2, B3, B6, and E as well as folate. With the exception of chestnuts—that have about 45 mg of vitamin C per serving—nuts aren't rich in vitamin C. In terms of vitamin E, almonds pack it in at 44 IU, followed by pine nuts at 16 IU, and peanuts at 13 IU per serving. The rest of the group don't have as much vitamin E. Hazelnuts and peanuts give you a generous dose of folate, at about 150 micrograms per serving, while the rest of the nuts in this group will give you 40 to 80 micrograms per serving.

These nuts will give you about 0.7 to 1.0 mg of vitamin B1 per serving, except for cashews that are a bit lower at 0.5 mg, and almonds, chestnuts, and walnuts fall behind at less than a quarter milligram. In terms of vitamin B2, almonds are the all-stars with 1.3 mg per serving, while chestnuts don't have much at all, and the rest fall at less than a quarter milligram per serving. A similar pattern holds for vitamin B3, where peanuts are the all-stars with 15 mg per serving, almonds are in second place with 4 mg per serving, and the rest fall behind at 2 or less milligrams per serving. In terms of vitamin B6, pistachios and pine nuts will give you nearly 2 mg per serving while the rest will give you only 0.2 to 0.7 mg per serving.

Beyond that, pecans and hazelnuts shine with the amount of bioflavonoids they pack—a whopping 500 mg or more per serving. Pistachios and pine nuts are not far behind at about 300 mg per serving. On average, they have about 20 to 30 mg of coenzyme Q10, and 40 to 70 mg of choline—you may remember from chapter 8 how wonderfully important this nutrient is for the retina and optic nerve. Peanuts have about 120 mg of choline per 4-ounce serving. The exception is that chestnuts and pistachios don't have much choline to talk about. Finally, pistachios and pine nuts have a generous 1.6 mg of lutein and zeaxanthin.

So as you see, these nuts have a tremendous variety of potent nutrients. Some are particularly strong in one category or another, but each one is an all-star. They are a good snack food and easy to take on the go. In addition, go ahead and use them for desserts or sprinkle them on your salad or entree.

BEANS

Beans are a tremendously valuable way to get your proteins and fiber all while stocking up on a whole host of nutrients. In fact, many doctors and nutritionists call them superfoods. This list of beans is by no means all inclusive—it's just meant to give you a taste of the nutritional values of the beans. Add beans to your meals once per day, either in an entree, as a side dish, or as a topping on a salad. They are best when cooked; some beans may even be toxic if uncooked or poorly cooked.

Black-Eyed Peas, Chickpeas, Edamame, Green Beans, Kidney Beans, Lentils, Lima Beans, Navy Beans, and White Beans

This collection of tasty seeds contains a nice balance of metal nutrients as well as phytic acid. Remember from our discussion in chapter 1 on oxidation that phytic acid helps balance out the metals by binding excess metals. While this enables it to bind the toxic metals, it can also bind good metals. However, these beans contain some of the good metals as well, and they do it in a balanced approach with the phytic acid to enable you to get a healthy amount of the metals you need.

This group of beans contain about 3 to 4 mg of phytic acid per 4-ounce serving, except for green beans, which contain less, at about 1 mg per serving. And that is fine that green beans contain less phytic acid, as they also have about half to a third of the metals that the other beans have. The other beans all have a good range of healthy metals: 3 to 4 mg of iron, 0.2 to 0.4 mg of copper, 1.1 to 1.7 mg of zinc, 40 to 70 mg of magnesium, and 0.5 to 1.1 mg of manganese per serving.

With their high protein content, these beans are also wonderful sources for those amino acids your body needs. Except for green beans, which are atypically low for this group—100 mg of arginine, 25 mg of methionine, 100 mg of lysine, and 75 mg of proline per serving—the others are nicely loaded with these amino acids. They have about 500 to 900 mg of arginine per serving, which will also afford you about 100 mg of methionine—except for white beans, which will support you with a bit more methionine, at 150 mg per serving. Each of the beans also has a nice dose of lysine—600 to 800 mg per serving—and of proline—400 to 600 mg per serving, except for edamame, which packs in the proline at 800 mg per serving.

Edamame is also the exception when it comes to choline, clocking in at 60 mg per 4-ounce serving, while the rest of the group rings in at 30 to 50 mg per serving. Green beans are again the weak link with only 20 mg per serving.

A similar pattern holds up with the lettered vitamins. Edamame nets you 350 micrograms of folate per serving, while the beans in the rest of the group get you about 100 to 200 micrograms of folate per serving. Green beans are again the weak link with only 40 micrograms per serving.

All the beans will get you 0.1 to 0.3 mg of vitamin B1, 0.1 to 0.2 mg of vitamin B2, 0.2 to 1.2 mg of vitamin B3, and 0.1 to 0.3 mg of vitamin B6 per serving. Navy beans top the list for B1, edamame for B2, edamame and lentils for B3 (with white beans down at the bottom), and chickpeas for B6. However, unlike the others, green beans will get you vitamin A—at 800 IU per serving.

FISH, MEAT, AND EGGS

This category fills the need for protein in most diets. Foods listed here often form the entree of the meal.

Meats

Unless you're a vegetarian, meats in moderation will get you three important nutrients: carnitine, which you can get to a lesser extent from milk and seafood; taurine, which is available in milk and seafood; and vitamin B12, which you can also obtain from seafood and to a lesser extent from eggs and milk. Eat meats in moderation, avoid extra oil and grease, and use beans and nuts to supplement your protein if you need to get more protein.

Eggs

Most people will want to get their eggs for breakfast, and that is certainly a reasonable breakfast meal—just stay light on the oil, depending on how you cook them. With a 4-ounce serving, you'll help yourself to a whopping 300 mg of choline! With that, you'll get a bit of vitamin A (600 IU), a bit of vitamin B2 (0.6 mg), a bit of vitamin D (60 IU), and only a trace of vitamin B12 (0.4 micrograms). While eggs have 2 mg of iron per serving, they also have nearly 40 micrograms of selenium per serving. Remember that we need to limit our selenium intake, but scientists believe that selenium from natural sources such as eggs is generally safe in this type of range. Of course, eggs will give you the protein-building blocks: arginine at 1,000 mg, methionine at 400 mg, lysine at 1,000 mg, and proline at 600 mg per serving. An egg or two a day is a wise choice for most people.

Fish: Salmon, Trout, Catfish, Flounder, Haddock, Sole, Shrimp, Anchovy, and Sardines

With all the health benefits of fish, a key concept is replacing meats with fish, and aiming for meats only in moderation and fish at least three or four times per week, if not more. The fish to avoid because of mercury are: mackerel, tuna, shark, swordfish, and rockfish. Other fish you may wish to avoid because of mercury levels (lower than the list above, but still too high) are cod, herring, and lobster. The "safe" fish in general are (in alphabetical order): anchovy, catfish, flounder, haddock, salmon, sardines, shrimp, sole, tilapia, and trout. The drawback with sardines and anchovy is that they are generally canned, they may be overly processed, and chemicals from the cans may leach into the foods.

We've talked a lot about the health benefits of DHA—the fish oil that helps from the front to the back of the eye—from dry eye to retinitis pigmentosa and macular degeneration. How much DHA do these types of fish have, and which one is the all-star? By far, the all-star is salmon, with 1,600 mg of DHA per 4-ounce serving! In distant second place is trout with 600 mg of DHA per serving. While anchovy also have 1,500 mg of DHA per serving and sardines 600 mg per serving, these two fish are not the go-to choices because they are canned. But if you need canned, then these two are the ones for you. The other fish on this list run at about 150 mg of DHA per serving.

While shrimp also has about 150 mg of DHA per serving, it is high in astaxanthin—the powerful antioxidant carotenoid that gives these shellfish their red color. Salmon and trout are also good choices for astaxanthin, particularly wild-caught salmon. Farm-raised salmon has astaxanthin added in its feed along with canthaxanthin, another carotenoid, used to "color" the salmon pink. However, while canthaxanthin is also an antioxidant, it can accumulate as crystals in the retina and may cause mild harm to the retina, though it often does not cause changes in vision. In addition, fish will afford you some glutathione and some alpha-lipoic acid, to top off your antioxidant warriors. It's best to go for fish baked or grilled, not fried.

GRAINS

Grains include fiber and carbohydrates and are an important part of a healthy diet. Grains have numerous health benefits, from prevention of heart disease to good digestive health, and may even help with weight loss—though because they are high in fiber, they will translate into starches that get slowly converted to sugars in the body, so diabetics must be cautious.

Whole grains are simply unrefined grains, while refined grains are processed to remove their bran (the covering husk) and germ (the small dense inner "nucleus" of the seed), which also removes many nutrients and leaves a very processed and polished by-product: white flour (used for white breads, cereals, crackers, desserts) or white rice. Some grains are then "enriched" or "fortified" by replacing nutrients that were lost or adding additional nutrients. However, the replacement is never like the original. Go for the whole grains. So with breakfast, lunch, and dinner, select healthy whole grains, in the form of breads, cereals, rice, or supplemental ingredients to your entree or side dish. A couple or more servings per day is a good goal for most people.

Just like beans, grains have some of the lettered vitamins, a varying amount of amino acids, as well as metals and phytic acid to balance the metals they contain and help us balance toxic metals we may consume in our diets. Unlike beans, grains do not contain folate.

Brown Rice

The various forms of brown rice are whole grains, unrefined with their dark and brown inner husk—the bran—still on the grain. All white rice is derived from brown rice and stripped of nutrients in the processing. In addition to the nutrients that are removed, bran oils—a healthy form of oil that may help in controlling cholesterol—is also lost. Go for the unrefined brown rice version of your favorite type of rice.

A 4-ounce serving of brown rice contains a splattering of helpful metals—0.5 mg of iron, 0.1 mg of copper, 0.7 mg of zinc, 55 mg of magnesium, and 1.0 mg of manganese. It also contains some B vitamins: 0.1 mg of B1, 1.7 mg of B3, and 0.2 mg of B6 per serving. A healthy serving of amino acids also come along for the ride: 700 mg of arginine, 200 mg of methionine, 350 mg of lysine, and 400 mg of proline. There is even a small amount of choline: 10 mg per serving.

Oatmeal and Granola

These grains can be added to breads or cereals or used for snacks. Oatmeal consists of one specific type of grain—an oat—that is ground or crushed, while granola is often a mixture of oat grains combined with nuts, dried fruits, and/or honey or sugar. The rolled oats are often processed to remove the bran, steamed, and then rolled flat, while steel-cut oats are often—though not always— unprocessed, just simply cut into smaller bits, to retain their bran. With both oatmeal and granola, go for the raw, whole grains, avoiding processed versions.

You'll get your metals: 3 to 5 mg of iron, 0.5 to 0.7 mg of copper, 3 to 5 mg of zinc, 100 to 200 mg of magnesium, and 3 to 5 mg of manganese per serving. Along with these nutrients, you'll be happy to obtain some B vitamins: 0.3 to 0.8 mg of B1, 0.1 to 0.3 mg of B2, 2.4 to 4.0 mg of B3, and 0.3 mg of B6. In addition to the typical splattering of amino acids—1,500 mg of arginine, 300 mg of methionine, 700 mg of lysine, and 900 mg of proline—you'll also get 30 to 60 mg of choline.

Flaxseed and Quinoa

These two delicious edible grains exhibit a slightly different nutritional profile than other grains. Flaxseed—also known as linseed—is a very small brown seed that looks like sesame seeds. Just like the oats above, it has a moderate amount of metals, lettered vitamins, amino acids, and choline. Unlike oats and other grains, flaxseed will get you a tremendous amount of omega-3 oil, though it's only one type of omega-3 oil—called ALA or alpha-linolenic acid—and it doesn't have any of the DHA omega-3 oil. It is also loaded with bioflavonoids, and it contains a phytochemical called lignin that serves as an antioxidant. However, use in moderation. A little bit goes a long way, and too much can have uncomfortable side effects such as abdominal discomfort or more serious gastrointestinal complications.

Quinoa comes from what is called the "goosefoot" family and originally came to us from the Andes mountain region of South America. It is quite versatile: It can be eaten raw or cooked, used in place of rice, or added to salads and soups. However, quinoa is often processed to remove its bitter outer layer, which contains a chemical that also irritates the gut. So keep in mind that quinoa is a refined grain, not a whole grain. Raw quinoa has a similar nutrient profile as oats, but unlike the other grains, quinoa will also get you some folate—over 200 micrograms worth in one 4-ounce serving. When cooked, though, it absorbs water, expands, and almost three-quarters of its weight is then water, which means its nutritional value drops by fourfold. Because it's a processed grain, use in moderation, as with flaxseed. A little bit is fine. Instead, go for the unprocessed whole grains.

FLAVORINGS AND SPICES

In various chapters we've discussed the health benefits of mint, saffron, curry, and garlic. We'll add cinnamon, basil, and ginger to that list. Go for them with your daily meals. And find your own favorites to add to this list.

Mint and Basil

These leafy flavorings can be used fresh—as whole leaf or chopped toppings—or cooked with meals to give them that extra zing. Mint and basil are both from the same family. In chapter 8 on glaucoma, we learned how mint is particularly potent in activating cell-signaling molecules that protect the neural cells of the eye. With its phytochemicals and numerous bioflavonoids, basil has numerous potent health benefits, from anti-inflammatory to antioxidant. Basil also has some special oils called "volatile oils" that are quite bioactive, especially helping against inflammation and protecting the cells in your eyes. In France, it is also known as the royal herb and its name comes from the Greek word for "royal." It and the other members of the mint family—oregano, lavender, sage, rosemary, thyme—certainly are royals when it comes to health.

In addition to these special nutrients, mint and basil will get you a few healthy grams of lutein and zeaxanthin as well as beta-carotene that translates to some 5,000 to 6,000 IU of vitamin A per 4-ounce serving. You'll get an assortment of other lettered vitamins such as a milligram or two of vitamin B3. There are some healthy essential metals: 4 to 6 mg of iron, a half milligram of copper, a milligram of zinc, some 70 to 90 mg of magnesium, and 1 to 1.5 mg of manganese. As with most leafy greens, you'll also end up with a hefty amount of vitamin K: up to 500 micrograms per serving.

Saffron

Derived from the flower of the saffron crocus plant, saffron has two uncommon carotenoids: crocin and crocetin, which are powerful antioxidants. In addition, it is quite potent with a whole host of other carotenoids: beta-carotene, lutein, and zeaxanthin—as well as many other nutrients, particularly vitamin C, at nearly 100 mg per 4 ounces and folate at over 100 micrograms per 4 ounces. Of course, with its light weight, you will only get a dab of it per dish, not the full 4-ounce serving. But it's an easy spice to add to rice and other dishes.

Curry

Curry is actually a mix of spices that contains curcumin, which comes from the ginger-like root of the turmeric plant. It has tremendous health benefits. Curry contains more than just the curcumin and curcuminoids—it has other minerals, lettered-vitamins, bioflavonoids, and choline. It packs a strong antioxidant punch and has anti-inflammatory as well as protective effects. It will provide a unique flavoring to your dishes.

Ginger

This flavoring is most closely related to curry. Cultivated from the root of the ginger plant, it contains bioactive compounds called gingerols that have been scientifically studied for their benefits in a wide variety of ailments of the body. While the verdict is still out for the most part, these gingerols are believed to be beneficial. Raw ginger contains the gingerols that, when cooked, get converted into different forms called zingerones and shogaols that have differing potencies and effects. So raw, pickled, or cooked, ginger may be a good spice to use.

Garlic

This "spice" belongs in the onion family and contains many of the same nutrients as onions, including about 25 mg of quercetin per serving. Garlic also has a compound called allicin, which we learned about in chapter 8 on glaucoma. While garlic is high in bioflavonoids, it is also high in selenium, but don't worry as you probably won't be eating a full 4-ounce serving all at once. Mix in some fresh garlic with your meals—in moderation—and you should receive the health benefits without the risks.

Cinnamon

With essential oils and other nutrients, the inner bark of this tree is often ground to a powdery form. This spice is packed with bioflavonoids: for comparison's sake, it has nearly 10,000 mg per 4-ounce serving! No, that was not a typo. It's in the same ballpark as cocoa beans and has nearly five times more bioflavonoids than its closest common-food competitor: dark, unsweetened chocolate, at up to 2,000 mg per 4-ounce serving. Of course, you probably won't eat 4 ounces of cinnamon all at once—and I certainly don't recommend that you do—but a single tablespoon mixed in your meal will get you over 600 mg of bioflavonoids.

Use it to flavor desserts, foods, coffees, and teas. It makes for a good topping on side dishes such as sweet potatoes or snacks and cereals. It can be used in powder form or in the form of cinnamon sticks. It's certainly a worthwhile flavoring to add to your daily rotation of flavors.

SWEETENERS

To sweeten up your desserts, coffees, and teas, avoid sugar, whether it is white refined sugar or brown sugar or turbinado—raw—sugar. While all these sugars are still "natural," brown sugar has a bit more molasses and raw sugar has perhaps a negligible trace of nutrients in it. Nevertheless, nearly six decades ago (in 1957), Dr. William Martin—a published medical researcher with an interest in nutrition—expressed his concerns about sugar and considered it a "poison."

And there is certainly an element of truth to his writings. Try to avoid foods with added sugars, as they will increase your risk of health problems, such as diabetes, heart and vascular disease, cancer, and Alzheimer's, and they will fill you up and decrease your appetite for other healthier options—instead of foods with added sugars, eat some more fruits and veggies, and load up on those healthy nutrients.

Honey

This sweet alternative to sugar is good in moderation. While honey still has the simple sugars in it that can cause the health concerns above, it is full of bioflavonoids from floral sources collected by the bees. However, the total quantity of bioflavonoids is a bit limited: perhaps only 1 to 2 mg per 4-ounce serving. More important than the quantity is the variety of floral bioflavonoids contained in honey, some perhaps quite potent. While it doesn't contain many of the nutrients we've discussed in this book, it does have small amounts of choline (2.5 mg). Overall, honey is certainly a good alternative to refined sugar, but that shouldn't give you permission to go overboard. The best advice is to limit these types of sugars, so that you have more room for fruits and veggies in your diet.

As a side note, keep in mind that honey should be avoided in pregnancy and in infants under the age of one because of toxins from bacteria that can grow in honey and cause botulism, a serious illness that often results in trouble breathing and paralysis. Older children and adults have protective mechanisms, so no worries with those over the age of one.

Figs and Dates

Alternatively, you can add small bits of figs and dates to sweeten your desserts or snacks. Go for the unsweetened dried figs or dates. Because they are fruits, they contain numerous other nutrients, such as bioflavonoids and choline. You'll also get a bit of iron and some other healthy metals—1 to 2 mg of iron, 0.2 to 0.3 mg of copper, 0.3 to 0.6 mg of zinc, 50 to 75 mg of magnesium, and 0.3 to 0.6 mg of manganese per serving—as well as some B vitamins. So if you can avoid sugar and sweeten with dried figs or dates, go for it!

Chocolate

You'll want unsweetened dark chocolate, and of course, unsweetened chocolate is not technically a sweetener! But it belongs in this category as a sweet-dish flavoring. Depending on the quality and origin, you'll get up to 2,000 mg—or perhaps a bit more—of bioflavonoids per 4-ounce serving. That goes a long way in your antioxidant armamentarium. It also affords you 50 mg of choline per serving as well as some amino acids: 900 mg of arginine, 150 mg of methionine, 500 mg of lysine, and 1,000 mg of proline per serving. With up to 3 mg of iron, 0.8 mg of copper, 2 mg of zinc, 130 mg of magnesium, and 1 mg of manganese per serving, there certainly is a nutritional benefit to unsweetened chocolate. Add to that some B vitamins—0.2 mg of B1, 0.1 mg of B2, and 1.5 mg of B3—and you're on your way to a nutritious day!

OILS

So you've heard from all sorts of places about the importance of oils that have less saturated fats for your overall health. But how much of a difference do these oils make for the eyes? There is no good data on the direct difference it makes, but indirectly by reducing cholesterol and reducing the risk of blood vessel disease (lumped in the category of heart-and-blood-vessel or cardiovascular disease, which also includes arteriosclerosis and atherosclerosis), you improve blood flow and oxygenation to your eyes.

You decrease the risk of diabetic retinopathy. You decrease the risk of glaucoma. You decrease the risk of having a stroke in the eye—and yes, just like you can get a stroke in the brain, you can get a stroke in the eye, where suddenly the blood flow to the eye's brain tissue—the retina—stops and the tissue gets injured sometimes temporarily and sometimes permanently, resulting in poor vision or blindness. You also decrease the risk of macular degeneration. We also learned about the debris that accumulates in macular degeneration, and high cholesterol, as we learned, is a risk factor for debris accumulating.

So which oils do you go for? The unsaturated vegetable oils. You've probably heard of all the benefits of olive oil. In addition, canola is a good basic vegetable oil. Flaxseed and walnut oils will provide you with omega-3 fatty acids. If you can, go for the cold-pressed oils, as they retain more of the nutrients in the oils, as well as providing you with more aroma and flavor.

Use these oils, but use them sparingly in your dishes. Avoid the other more saturated fats and oils. As we've discussed repeatedly throughout the book, you do need some oils—a small amount—to help absorb the fat-soluble vitamins, and you do need your omega-3 and omega-6 oils in a balanced approach.

DRINKS

It goes without saying: Get rid of the sodas and sugary drinks! Don't go for the diet sodas either, because there is a growing body of evidence about the health risks of drinking them. So what does that leave you with? Water, milk, tea, coffee, and 100 percent pure fruit juice.

Water and Fruit Juice

Water of course quenches your thirst and replenishes your fluid levels in your body. Generally speaking, it is missing electrolytes and nutritional value, but that certainly does not diminish its value. Fruit juice, on the other hand, is full of nutritional value, predominantly from the fruits from which it is derived. It is a good alternative to obtaining your daily fruit requirement, if you're not able to eat the fruits otherwise. Go for fresh-squeezed juice. Feel free to mix juice and water to add flavor to the water or lighten up the juice.

Tea and Coffee

Coffee will get you bioflavonoids as well as some B vitamins. However, tea is really the all-star in this category. Teas will get you hundreds of milligrams of bioflavonoids per cup—and with many different varieties, you'll end up with many different types of bioflavonoids. Whether you prefer caffeinated or decaffeinated—herbal or green, white, or black—aim for a cup or two or three a day, scattered through the day!

Milk

It was our favorite drink—and meal—right after we were born, and it is a good choice, full of essential nutrients for your eyes and vision, as well as proteins and calcium for your muscles and bones. We all know that milk has vitamin D—about 100 IU per cup—which is essential for the eye's immune defense as well as signaling in the neurons of the retina and optic nerve.

Beyond that, with its protein content, it has some of the important amino acids for collagen formation (lysine and proline), for blood flow (arginine), for energy boosting and debris removal (methionine and carnitine), and for prevention of retinal disease, diabetes, and cataracts (taurine, which is one of the most concentrated amino acids in the retina). Remember that the main sources for taurine are meats, but milk and seaweed also have it to a lesser extent. The same holds for carnitine, which is predominantly in meat, but also to a lesser extent in dairy products.

Milk also has some B vitamins, including vitamin B12, which is essential for protection of DNA and insulation of your nerves, including your two optic nerves. Milk will get you along your way to a minimum of 5 micrograms per day with its 1 to 1.25 micrograms of vitamin B12 per cup. A cup or two a day will go a long way!

SAMPLE MEAL PLANS

So we've gone through quite a few categories of foods in our healthy vision menu. How do you put it all together in daily meal plan format? Here is a sample meal plan:

Breakfast
Go for eggs and add whole grains. Sparingly use unsaturated oils. You can use honey, or better yet some dried figs or dates—or even a fresh fruit compote without added sugars—to sweeten your whole grain toast or whole grain cereal. Take the opportunity to get a serving or two of fruits into your meal, or perhaps even some veggies.

Lunch or Dinner Entree
Fish should be included in your rotation at least several times per week. A wonderful daily selection is salad with some of the all-star veggie ingredients: spinach, kale, red cabbage, parsley, tomatoes, onions, corn, peppers, mushrooms, broccoli sprouts, and avocado. Add some mint or basil to your daily salad, and certainly look at adding beans or nuts too. A little of the unsaturated oils can serve as a healthy dressing. When eating sandwiches, use whole grain breads. In entrees, go for healthy flavorings and spices such as saffron, curry, garlic, ginger, and basil.

Lunch or Dinner Side Dishes

You'll certainly want to include vegetables as your side-dish options. Sweet potatoes are an excellent option several times per week. Other top choices include squash, brussels sprouts, and asparagus, as well as other veggies from the categories we've talked about in the beginning of this chapter—or find and choose your own favorites. Certainly include beans—the many different types—and grains, particularly whole grain brown rice, several times per week.

Snacks and Desserts

Fruits should really be the mainstay of most people's snacks and desserts—of course, diabetics should take caution. Adding fruits several times per day is extremely beneficial for your eyes and vision. As an alternative to fruits, veggies can be included in the snack mix, with broccoli and carrots as top munchies choices—with a tiny dab of dip.

Nuts are also a good choice as a stand-alone snack or a topping to a fruit-based dessert. Sweet potatoes or pumpkin is a good veggie for dessert. A no-sugar-added fruit compote is a healthy choice as a topping to a dessert. As a healthy snack, air-popped popcorn will afford you most of the nutrients of corn.

Flavorings such as mint, ginger, and cinnamon are nutritious choices for your desserts. Lightly sweeten your desserts with fruits or dried figs and dates, and a bit of honey instead of sugar. Milk chocolate and sweetened dark chocolate are not the best choices, but if you can satisfy your chocolate craving with lightly sweetened or unsweetened desserts that include unsweetened dark chocolate, it is chock-full of health benefits.

Drinks

Tea and milk are the top go-to choices for your daily regimen. Water, fruit juice, and coffee are also part of the mix.

• • •

As you and I and the research community learn more about various foods and their nutritional benefits, let's keep expanding our list. Don't forget to add your favorites and don't limit yourself. Make healthy choices! Talk to your doctor about your specific needs—there's no one size that fits all. With these suggestions, you should be well on your way to a "healthy vision" lifestyle.

CONCLUSION:
BUILDING THE RIGHT TEAM

Throughout *Healthy Vision* I hope that I have shown you how nutrition can help alleviate eye conditions and prevent vision loss. Eating the right nutrients is like building a great sports or professional team: You need people with different skills, who complement each other and work together to create a balanced approach and the best results. Having just one top-notch player on your team may not be enough to make it to the championship. Having a balanced, healthy diet rich in nutrients works the same way.

And nutrients do interact with each other. Let's take for example some specific foods such as blueberries, black currants, brussels sprouts, and red cabbage. These foods all contain wonderful nutrients, particularly antioxidant nutrients. But they also all contain chemicals called polyhydroxyphenols that can inactivate vitamin B1. Remember, we need vitamin B1 for energy production and neural signaling. So should we avoid these foods? What can we do? Well it turns out that including vitamin C and citric acid in one's diet can help block the ability of polyhydroxyphenols to inactive vitamin B1—it all gets balanced out with . . . a *balanced* nutritional program.

And we remember from chapter 1 on antioxidants that alpha-lipoic acid acts with vitamin C, vitamin E, bioflavonoids, and glutathione to form a highly protective antioxidant team. Alpha-lipoic acid and vitamin C protect glutathione from being used up. In turn, glutathione assists vitamin E and recycles vitamin C.

Balance is also essential because sometimes nutrients compete with each other. For example, it is important to note that beta-carotene can compete with lutein for absorption in the digestive tract, so that excess beta-carotene can result in lutein deficiency.

While high amounts of beta-carotene can decrease lutein absorption, high amounts of lutein do not decrease beta-carotene absorption.

Sometimes it's a delicate balance with any one given nutrient. We learned how metals can perform essential functions within our cells, but if we have too much of them, they can act as toxic oxidants. The same with methionine—it acts as an antioxidant, but if there's too much methionine, it gets converted to that toxic joker homocysteine that causes all that damage within cells we learned about in chapter 4.

We saw this theme throughout the book: vitamin B2 is required for activation of folate and vitamin B6; vitamin B12 deficiency results in folate deficiency; vitamin C increases intake of iron; excess iron may prevent the normal transport of chromium; and we could go on for pages.

And did you think that you should have your nutrients all in a fat-free diet? No! You need some fats. That's why they're in our diets. But it needs to be balanced . . . not too much. Let's take the carotenoids again. Digestion of fruits and vegetables occurs in the stomach with the assistance of stomach acids that help break down the fruits and vegetables to release the carotenoids. The carotenoids are not soluble in water, and so they need to be dissolved in fat micelles (spherical soap-bubble-like conglomerates of fat) that can carry the carotenoids into the bloodstream from the intestines. Accordingly, eating a small quantity of fat with the carotenoids assists in the absorption of the carotenoids and greatly increases the amount that is delivered to the bloodstream.

Interact, recycle, build the best nutrient team! Nutrients interact with each other. Nutrients recycle each other.

And finally, nutrition is for everyone, including those with good health and no eye problems. Even if you're not thinking about prevention right now, nutrition can help you now. Just recently, a small clinical trial showed that—in healthy people with absolutely no eye conditions—taking DHA (fish oil) for ninety days resulted in improvements in their ability to see! It only took ninety days, and these healthy people could see better! However, it was only a slight improvement, and the study was very small, making it more along the lines of preliminary report that warrants further studies rather than a definitive report. Nevertheless, the message is that nutrition is really for everyone: for those in good health, to prevent disease and optimize health, and for those already with eye conditions to help prevent worsening.

Nutrients are indeed the tools to improve the functioning of our cells. It's time to get to eating healthy foods!

APPENDIX: PRESCRIPTION FOR YOUR PLATE

This section is the go-to guide for readers who have been diagnosed with a disease, have noticed that their vision just keeps getting weaker every time they visit their eye doctor, or who simply want to avoid developing glaucoma like Grandma.

Each category of nutrients has its own section, all related to the six major conditions we discussed in Part II of the book. I provide a general guide to how much of each nutrient to target and what foods will get you on your way to your goals.

This appendix contains a massive amount of scientific information and medical research, organized in summaries and charts correlating more than fifty nutrients and the eye conditions they help. It serves as both a recipe and a reference to readers, so you can take aim at a condition or disease with the foods you eat. Here are specifics for certain conditions:

MACULAR DEGENERATION

For those who want to protect against macular degeneration or who have macular degeneration and want to reduce the risk of progression, the core nutrients are essential: the bioflavonoids, the carotenoids, the antioxidants, and the essential lettered vitamins. Don't overdo any of the nutrients, particularly the lettered vitamins. Take care with vitamin B2 because of its photosensitivity risks. The metals must also be taken in balance. Additional nutrients to obtain include phytic acid, carnitine, and omega-3 oils.

RETINITIS PIGMENTOSA

For those who want to protect against progression of retinitis pigmentosa, the core nutrients are essential: the bioflavonoids, the carotenoids, the antioxidants, and the essential lettered vitamins. Don't overdo any of the nutrients, particularly the lettered vitamins. Take care with vitamin B2 because of its photosensitivity risks. The metals must also be taken in balance. Additional nutrients to obtain include coenzyme Q10, mint, curry, and omega-3 oils.

DIABETIC RETINOPATHY

For those who want to protect against diabetic retinopathy, the core nutrients are essential: the bioflavonoids, the carotenoids, the antioxidants, and the essential lettered vitamins. Don't overdo any of the nutrients, particularly the lettered vitamins and the proteins. The metals must also be taken in balance, with limits on chromium and vanadium. Additional nutrients to obtain include agaricus, mint, and curry.

GLAUCOMA

For those who want to protect against development of glaucoma or who have glaucoma and want to reduce the risk of progression, the core nutrients are essential: the bioflavonoids, the carotenoids, the antioxidants, and the essential lettered vitamins. Don't overdo any of the nutrients, particularly the lettered vitamins. The metals must also be taken in balance, with care to avoid excess selenium. Additional nutrients to obtain include coenzyme Q10, choline, mint, proline, and lysine.

CATARACTS

For those who want to protect against development of cataracts or who have cataracts and want to reduce the risk of progression, the core nutrients are essential: the bioflavonoids, the carotenoids, the antioxidants, and the essential lettered vitamins. Don't overdo any of the nutrients, particularly the lettered vitamins. Take care with vitamin B2 because of its photosensitivity risks. The metals must also be taken in balance. Overall, of all the nutrients, the lettered nutrients are particularly important.

DRY EYE

For those who want to protect against and treat dry eye, the core nutrients are essential: the bioflavonoids, the carotenoids, the antioxidants, and the essential lettered vitamins. Don't overdo any of the nutrients, particularly the lettered vitamins, but make sure to get sufficient supply of vitamin A and vitamin C. The metals must also be taken in balance. Additional nutrients to include are the omega-3 and omega-6 oils, which must be appropriately balanced.

• • •

The following charts include the core nutrients that are—in general—helpful to all: bioflavonoids, carotenoids, unique plant nutrients, the super-antioxidants, metals and a metalloid, the lettered vitamins, amino acids, the special power nutrients, and fish oils. *Values in parentheses are commonly reported average amounts found in a 4-ounce serving size, except for coffee, tea, and milk, which are for an 8-ounce cup.*

Important Note: The recommended daily doses listed in the following tables are general, approximated guidelines based on reviews of multiple sources and are not intended as medical advice. Doses will vary from person to person depending on health status and health condition. Consult your doctor for guidelines and doses that are appropriate for you.

BIOFLAVONOIDS

This group contains thousands of nutrients found in plants that often act as powerful antioxidants. There are no established clear guidelines on how much to take because they are simply non-essential, and in fact the human body absorbs little of the bioflavonoids we eat. Some of the best sources are:

Fruits		Vegetables	
blueberries (400 mg)		parsley (270 mg)	
plums (280 mg)		red cabbage (200 mg)	
blackberries (200 mg)		kale (100 mg)	
peaches (100 mg)		peppermint leaves (70 mg)	
cherries (80 mg)		red onions (60 mg)	
grapes (60 mg)		red chile peppers (45 mg)	
lemons (60 mg)		okra (25 mg)	
red raspberries (50 mg)		broccoli (15 mg)	
strawberries (50 mg)		spinach (15 mg)	
oranges (50 mg)		romaine lettuce (5 mg)	
grapefruit (40 mg)			
pears (25 mg)		Beans	black-eyed peas (330 mg)
apricots (20 mg)			black beans (30 mg)
bananas (20 mg)			pinto beans (6 mg)
apples (15 mg)			green beans (4 mg)
tomatoes (2 mg)			
		Other	cocoa beans (9,900 mg)
Nuts	pecans (500 mg)		dark unsweetened chocolate (2,000 mg)
	hazelnuts (500 mg)		green tea (310 mg)
	pistachios (300 mg)		black tea (270 mg)
	pine nuts (300 mg)		bee pollen (30 mg)

Diindolylmethane—DIM

This bioflavonoid controls inflammation. Some of the best sources are:

Vegetables	broccoli	kale
	cauliflower	bok choy
	brussels sprouts	watercress
	cabbage	

Quercetin

This bioflavonoid is a powerful antioxidant and controls inflammation. Some of the best sources are:

Vegetables	red chile peppers (40 mg)	Fruits	plums (7 mg)
	red onions (40 mg)		blueberries (6 mg)
	okra (30 mg)		pears (5 mg)
	kale (10 mg)		apples (3 mg)
	romaine lettuce (5 mg)		cherries (3 mg)
	spinach (5 mg)		apricots (2 mg)
	green beans (4 mg)		strawberries (1 mg)
	broccoli (3 mg)		
		Nuts	pistachios (2 mg)
Beans	black-eyed peas (20 mg)		
		Other	bee pollen (24 mg)
			green tea (6 mg)
			black tea (5 mg)

Resveratrol

This bioflavonoid has strong antioxidant and anti-cancer activity. Its sources are limited, particularly to the skin of the muscadine grape.

Troxerutin

This bioflavonoid improves circulation. Some of the best sources are:

Fruit	citrus	Vegetables	asparagus
	apples (particularly the peels)		green peppers
	peaches		
	apricots	Grains	buckwheat
	raw cranberries		

CAROTENOIDS

The carotenoids are organic plant pigments that serve antioxidant and other roles.

Astaxanthin

This sea carotenoid is a powerful antioxidant. Some of the best sources are:

Fish   krill
                  shrimp
                  salmon
                  trout
Vegetables   algae

Beta-Carotene

This antioxidant carotenoid is the "orange" carotenoid, found in orange-colored vegetables and fruits, as well as some green- and red-colored vegetables and fruits in which the green or red color overpowers the orange pigment hidden inside. A daily consumption of 2 mg or less is often sufficient, but most people should aim to get 10 to 15 mg per day. While it is safe to go up to as much as 300 mg per day, you probably don't want or need to exceed 30 mg per day. However, in smokers, 20 mg per day or more may be unsafe because it has been found to increase the risk of lung cancer in smokers. Some of the best sources are:

Vegetables sweet potatoes (12 mg)   **Fruits**   cantaloupe (3 mg)
                kale (10 mg)   apricots (1 mg)
                carrots (9 mg)   mangoes (1 mg)
                spinach (7 mg)   pink grapefruit (1 mg)
                collard greens (6 mg)
                pumpkin (6 mg)
                parsley (5 mg)
                romaine lettuce (4 mg)
                squash (3 mg)
                red peppers (2 mg)

Crocin and Crocetin

These carotenoids are powerful antioxidants. They come from saffron.

Lutein and Zeaxanthin

These carotenoids—"yellow" ones—are powerful antioxidants found in yellow and orange vegetables as well as in green vegetables that also contain the yellow pigment hidden inside. Daily consumption of 6 to 12 mg is often a good target amount for lutein. Zeaxanthin can be made from lutein by the cells within the retina. Nevertheless, a daily consumption of 4 to 8 mg is often a good target amount for zeaxanthin. Some of the best sources are:

Vegetables	kale (23 mg)	brussels sprouts (2 mg)
	spinach (15 mg)	corn (1 mg)
	parsley (6 mg)	green beans (1 mg)
	green peas (3 mg)	pumpkin (1 mg)
	romaine lettuce (3 mg)	scallions (1 mg)
	squash (3 mg)	okra (0.5 mg)
	broccoli (2 mg)	red chile peppers (0.5 mg)

Lycopene

This antioxidant carotenoid is the "red" carotenoid, found in some red- and pink-colored fruits and vegetables. A daily consumption of 4 to 8 mg is often a good target amount for lycopene. Some of the best sources are:

Vegetables	tomatoes (3 mg)

Fruits	guava (6 mg)
	watermelon (5 mg)
	grapefruit (2 mg)
	papaya (2 mg)

UNIQUE PLANT NUTRIENTS

This group contains plant-derived nutrients.

Agaricus

This nutrient is potent against inflammation. There are no established clear guidelines on how much to take because it is simply non-essential. This nutrient comes from the white button pizza mushroom and the portobello mushroom.

Curcumin

Turmeric contains a biologically powerful agent called curcumin. There are no established clear guidelines on how much to take because it is simply non-essential. This nutrient is commonly found in curry powder, which contains turmeric.

Gingko

This is an antioxidant and anti–blood clotting nutrient. There are no established clear guidelines on how much to take because it is simply non-essential. Because it increases the risk of bleeding, daily dosages should probably be limited to around 30 mg per day, and certainly should not exceed 250 mg per day. This nutrient comes from the gingko biloba tree.

Mint Coleus

This nutrient increases signaling molecules within cells. There are no established clear guidelines on how much to take because it is simply non-essential, and it is believed that the human body absorbs little of the mint coleus we eat. This nutrient comes from the coleus mint plant.

Phytic Acid

This plant nutrient binds toxic metals and removes them from action, as well as removing debris from the retina. Because it can bind metals, it can also bind metals that the body needs, resulting in a deficiency in those metals. Therefore excess phytic should be avoided during pregnancy and in children. A typical healthy diet with a wide array of vegetables often will not exceed or even come close to reaching detrimental levels. Some of the best sources are:

Vegetables	spinach (4 mg)	**Nuts**	Brazil nuts (2 mg)
	carrots (3 mg)		almonds (1.5 mg)
	olives (3 mg)		walnuts (1 mg)
	beets (2 mg)		
	mushrooms (2 mg)	**Grains**	wild rice (1 mg)
	scallions (2 mg)		whole wheat bread (0.5 mg)
	cauliflower (1 mg)		whole wheat pasta (0.5 mg)
	broccoli (1 mg)		
	potatoes (1 mg)	**Other**	soybean tofu (4 mg)
	sweet potatoes (1 mg)		
Beans	kidney beans (4 mg)		
	lentils (4 mg)		
	navy beans (3 mg)		
	white beans (3 mg)		
	chickpeas (3 mg)		
	black-eyed peas (3 mg)		
	green beans (1 mg)		

St. John's Wort

This herb blocks inflammation and growth of abnormal blood vessels. There are no established clear guidelines on how much to take because it is simply non-essential. Because it increases the risk of light-toxicity reactions (see chapter 3), daily dosages should probably be limited to around 300 mg per day at most. Not everyone needs or should take St. John's Wort.

THE SUPER-ANTIOXIDANTS

Alpha-Lipoic Acid

This is the antioxidant of antioxidants. A daily consumption of 200 to 600 mg per day is often recommended. Since food sources often contain lower amounts, taking supplements—spread out in multiple doses throughout the day—may be a reasonable way to increase consumption. Care should be taken in diabetics, as it may lower blood sugars, in some cases to critically low levels. Some of the best sources are:

Meats/Dairy		Vegetables	
steak (0.3 mg)		spinach (0.2 mg)	
chicken (0.1 mg)		broccoli (0.1 mg)	
fish (0.1 mg)		peas (0.05 mg)	
eggs (0.1 mg)		brussels sprouts (0.05 mg)	
		tomatoes (0.05 mg)	

Glutathione

This antioxidant is involved in several other important activities. There are no established clear guidelines on how much to take. A normal healthy liver already produces about 13,000 mg of glutathione per day. Most people should aim to supplement that with anywhere from 100 up to 600 additional mg per day, from natural sources as there is some evidence that supplementation in the form of pills is often ineffective. Some of the best sources are:

Nuts			
walnuts (17 mg)		green peppers (6 mg)	
		green peas (6 mg)	
Meat/Fish		cucumbers (5 mg)	
ground beef (20 mg)		turnip greens (4 mg)	
steak (15 mg)			
chicken (15 mg)			
cod (7 mg)	**Fruits**	avocados (32 mg)	
pollock (3 mg)		tomatoes (10 mg)	
tuna (2 mg)		lemons (10 mg)	
shrimp (1.5 mg)		peaches (9 mg)	
		grapefruit (9 mg)	
Vegetables		oranges (8 mg)	
asparagus (33 mg)		strawberries (8 mg)	
potatoes (16 mg)		watermelon (8 mg)	
spinach (14 mg)		cantaloupe (8 mg)	
okra (14 mg)		papaya (7 mg)	
squash (13 mg)		mangoes (6 mg)	
cauliflower (11 mg)		pears (6 mg)	
broccoli (10 mg)		apples (4 mg)	
carrots (9 mg)			
red peppers (8 mg)			

Sulforaphane

This plant chemical is a tremendous antioxidant and anti-cancer agent. There are no established clear guidelines on how much to take because it is simply non-essential. Nevertheless, because of its utility, most people should aim to get in 50 to 400 micrograms per day when possible. Sources are:

Vegetable   baby broccoli sprouts (300 micrograms)
broccoli spears (20 micrograms)
brussels sprouts (9 micrograms)
red cabbage (6 micrograms)
cabbage (3 micrograms)
cauliflower (3 micrograms)

METALS AND A METALLOID

While some metals are essential for good health, remember to monitor amounts closely to avoid harmful effects.

Boron

This element is the metalloid in the group. It maintains hormonal balance and enhances the activity of many enzymes. The often recommended daily allowance of boron is 500 to 3,000 micrograms per day. Some of the best sources are:

Vegetables	broccoli (290 micrograms)	**Fruits**	peaches (610 micrograms)
	carrots (260 micrograms)		grapes (560 micrograms)
	onions (220 micrograms)		apples (410 micrograms)
	spinach (210 micrograms)		pears (320 micrograms)
	potatoes (130 micrograms)		oranges (300 micrograms)
	lettuce (120 micrograms)		cantaloupe (210 micrograms)
	corn (50 micrograms)		bananas (160 micrograms)
			tomatoes (70 micrograms)
Beans	black-eyed peas (530 micrograms)		
	lima beans (430 micrograms)		
	peas (150 micrograms)		
	string beans (140 micrograms)		
	black beans (40 micrograms)		

Chromium

This metal may regulate insulin and remove debris from the retina. The reasonable balanced amount of chromium for most people is between 50 and 100 micrograms per day. Some of the best sources are:

Vegetables	broccoli (22 micrograms)	**Dairy**	cheese (0.6 microgram)
	potatoes (3 micrograms)		eggs (0.2 microgram)
	green beans (2 micrograms)		
	lettuce (2 micrograms)	**Meats**	haddock (100 micrograms)
			steak (2 micrograms)
Fruits	tomatoes (1 microgram)		turkey breast (2 micrograms)
	apples (1 microgram)		chicken breast (0.5 microgram)
	bananas (1 microgram)		
Grains	wheat bread (5 micrograms)		
	white rice (1 microgram)		

Copper

This antioxidant metal can also act as an oxidant. It also activates many genes and is essential for many enzymes. The reasonable balanced amount of copper for most people is between 2 to 3 mg per day. The amount of copper should be titrated with zinc to achieve a tenfold zinc amount compared to copper. Careful with copper if you are prone to high cholesterol, as it may increase cholesterol levels. Some of the best sources are:

Meat/Fish	lobster (2.2 mg)	**Beans**	chickpeas (0.4 mg)
	crab (1.3 mg)		edamame (0.4 mg)
	shrimp (0.3 mg)		black-eyed peas (0.3 mg)
	steak (0.1 mg)		lentils (0.3 mg)
			lima beans (0.3 mg)
Nuts	cashews (2.5 mg)		white beans (0.3 mg)
	sunflower seeds (2.1 mg)		kidney beans (0.2 mg)
	hazelnuts (2.0 mg)		navy beans (0.2 mg)
	pine nuts (1.5 mg)		green beans (0.1 mg)
	pistachios (1.5 mg)		
	walnuts (1.5 mg)	**Fruits**	avocados (2.1 mg)
	pecans (1.4 mg)		dried figs (0.3 mg)
	almonds (1.3 mg)		dates (0.2 mg)
	peanuts (1.0 mg)		
	chestnuts (0.5 mg)	**Other**	chocolate (0.8 mg)
			soy milk (0.3 mg)
Vegetables	avocado (2.1 mg)		tofu (0.2 mg)
	mushrooms (0.4 mg)		
	basil (0.4 mg)	**Grains**	raw flaxseed (1.4 mg)
	mint (0.4 mg)		raw granola (0.7 mg)
	artichokes (0.3 mg)		raw quinoa (0.6 mg)
	potatoes (0.2 mg)		raw oatmeal (0.5 mg)
	spinach (0.2 mg)		wild brown rice (0.1 mg)
	sweet potatoes (0.2 mg)		

Iron

In addition to its role in carrying oxygen in red blood cells, iron is essential for hundreds of enzymes and proteins. Iron doses vary by age and by gender and during pregnancy. For most adults, a reasonable dose is 10 to 15 mg per day. Some of the best sources are:

Meat/Fish	steak (3 mg)	**Fruits**	dried figs (2 mg)
	lean ground beef (3 mg)		dates (1 mg)
	lamb (2 mg)		
	shrimp (1.5 mg)	**Beans**	lentils (4 mg)
	dark meat chicken (1.5 mg)		white beans (4 mg)
	white meat chicken (1.0 mg)		black-eyed peas (3 mg)
			chickpeas (3 mg)
			edamame (3 mg)
Grains	raw flaxseed (6 mg)		kidney beans (3 mg)
	raw granola (5 mg)		lima beans (3 mg)
	raw quinoa (5 mg)		navy beans (3 mg)
	raw oatmeal (3 mg)		green beans (1 mg)
	rice (3 mg)		
	cornbread (2 mg)	**Nuts**	almonds (6 mg)
	white bread (2 mg)		cashews (6 mg)
			chestnuts (6 mg)
Vegetables	mint (6 mg)		hazelnuts (6 mg)
	basil (4 mg)		peanuts (6 mg)
	spinach (4 mg)		pecans (6 mg)
	carrots (3 mg)		pine nuts (6 mg)
	olives (3 mg)		pistachios (6 mg)
	beets (2 mg)		walnuts (6 mg)
	mushrooms (2 mg)		
	scallions (2 mg)	**Other**	tofu (4 mg)
	cauliflower (1 mg)		chocolate (3 mg)
	potatoes (1 mg)		eggs (2 mg)
	sweet potatoes (1 mg)		

Magnesium

This metal activates many enzymes including those for energy. Recommended doses vary by age, but a good rule of thumb is to balance it around 300 to 420 mg per day. Some of the best sources are:

Nuts
almonds (300 mg)
cashews (300 mg)
hazelnuts (200 mg)
peanuts (200 mg)
walnuts (200 mg)
pecans (140 mg)
pine nuts (140 mg)
pistachios (140 mg)
chestnuts (30 mg)

Grains
raw flaxseed (450 mg)
raw granola (200 mg)
raw quinoa (200 mg)
raw oatmeal (130 mg)
brown rice (55 mg)

Meat/Fish
crab (970 mg)
sole (65 mg)
shrimp (50 mg)
lobster (40 mg)
salmon (35 mg)
cod (35 mg)
chicken (30 mg)

Dairy
yogurt (40 mg)
swiss cheese (40 mg)
milk (20 mg)

Vegetables
spinach (100 mg)
mint (90 mg)
artichoke (70 mg)
basil (70 mg)

Fruits
dried figs (75 mg)
dates (50 mg)

Beans
edamame (70 mg)
white beans (70 mg)
black-eyed peas (60 mg)
navy beans (60 mg)
chickpeas (50 mg)
kidney beans (50 mg)
lima beans (50 mg)
lentils (40 mg)
green beans (20 mg)

Other
espresso (190 mg)
unsweetened chocolate powder
 (130 mg)
coffee (7 mg)

Manganese

This metal is also an essential metal for many enzymes. The most often recommended dose allowance is 3 to 5 mg per day. Some of the best sources are:

Nuts	hazelnuts (7.0 mg)	**Beans**	chickpeas (1.1 mg)
	pecans (5.1 mg)		edamame (1.1 mg)
	walnuts (4.4 mg)		white beans (0.7 mg)
	almonds (2.5 mg)		lima beans (0.6 mg)
	peanuts (2.1 mg)		navy beans (0.6 mg)
	cashews (1.8 mg)		black-eyed peas (0.5 mg)
	chestnuts (1.4 mg)		kidney beans (0.5 mg)
	pine nuts (1.4 mg)		lentils (0.5 mg)
	pistachios (1.4 mg)		
		Vegetables	basil (1.3 mg)
Fruits	coconut (1.7 mg)		mint (1.3 mg)
	pineapple (1.4 mg)		spinach (1.0 mg)
	raspberries (0.8 mg)		collard greens (0.5 mg)
	dried figs (0.6 mg)		kale (0.5 mg)
	dates (0.3 mg)		
		Other	unsweetened chocolate powder
Grains	raw granola (4.6 mg)		(1.0 mg)
	raw oatmeal (3.0 mg)		green tea (0.5 mg)
	wheat bread (3.0 mg)		black tea (0.4 mg)
	raw flaxseed (2.8 mg)		
	raw quinoa (2.0 mg)		
	brown rice (1.0 mg)		

Selenium

While it is essential for certain enzymes, this metal is also a toxic oxidant. The minimum recommended amount is 55 micrograms per day, and most people can go up to 100 micrograms per day. There is a risk of glaucoma at levels of 200 micrograms per day. So use caution when selecting foods—a 4 ounce serving of Brazil nuts, for example, will take you well over that limit! Some of the best sources are:

Fruits
dates (3 micrograms)
dried figs (0.7 micrograms)

Nuts
Brazil nuts (2,200 micrograms)
sunflower seeds
(90 micrograms)
walnuts (6 micrograms)

Meat/Fish
sole (66 micrograms)
cod (53 micrograms)
lobster (48 micrograms)
shrimp (47 micrograms)
crab (45 micrograms)
salmon (43 micrograms)
steak (39 micrograms)
chicken breast (32 micrograms)
dark meat chicken
(23 micrograms)

Dairy
eggs (37 micrograms)
ricotta cheese (17 micrograms)
cottage cheese (12 micrograms)
milk (9 micrograms)

Vegetables
mushrooms (11 micrograms)

Grains
raw oatmeal (50 micrograms)
wheat bread (47 micrograms)
raw flaxseed (30 micrograms)
raw granola (30 micrograms)
white bread (36 micrograms)
brown rice (10 micrograms)
raw quinoa (8 micrograms)

Vanadium

This metal can help in diabetes and decrease cholesterol and lower blood pressure, but it causes oxidative damage. The amount that is likely safe is around 25 to 50 micrograms per day, and probably higher when obtained through natural sources; through pills, it is probably best not to exceed 100 micrograms per day. In other words, a healthy, balanced diet will likely get you much more than 100 micrograms per day, but that is believed to be acceptable and healthy when obtained through natural sources—so in that case there is no need to supplement it with pills, as the toxicity is believed to arise when vanadium is supplemented by pills. Some of the best sources are:

Beans	lentils (690 micrograms)	Fruits	tangerines (20 micrograms)
	navy beans (590 micrograms)		avocado (10 micrograms)
	green peas (380 micrograms)		
		Nuts	hazelnuts (220 micrograms)
Vegetables	alfalfa (460 micrograms)		pecans (90 micrograms)
	radishes (350 micrograms)		walnuts (30 micrograms)
	parsley (210 micrograms)		
	cabbage (200 micrograms)	Dairy	eggs (53 micrograms)
	potatoes (170 micrograms)		
	squash (140 micrograms)	Meats/Fish	lobster (590 micrograms)
	lettuce (120 micrograms)		scallops (240 micrograms)
	carrots (110 micrograms)		cod (110 micrograms)
	spinach (60 micrograms)		chicken breast (20 micrograms)
	corn (60 micrograms)		

Zinc

This essential metal plays a role in hundreds of enzymes and is needed for making DNA. The reasonable balanced amount of zinc for most people is between 20 to 30 mg per day. The amount of copper should be titrated with copper to achieve a tenfold zinc amount compared to copper. Careful with copper if you are prone to high cholesterol, as it may increase cholesterol levels. Some of the best sources are:

Meat/Fish
crab (8.6 mg)
ground beef (7.1 mg)
steak (6.2 mg)
lobster (3.3 mg)
dark meat chicken (3.3 mg)
shrimp (1.6 mg)
chicken breast (1.1 mg)
sole (0.7 mg)
cod (0.6 mg)
salmon (0.6 mg)

Nuts
cashews (6.5 mg)
pecans (5.1 mg)
peanuts (3.8 mg)
walnuts (3.8 mg)
almonds (3.5 mg)
hazelnuts (2.8 mg)
pine nuts (2.5 mg)
pistachios (2.5 mg)
chestnuts (1.0 mg)

Dairy
swiss cheese (5.0 mg)
provolone cheese (3.7 mg)
cheddar cheese (3.5 mg)
muenster cheese (3.2 mg)
yogurt (2.0 mg)
eggs (1.3 mg)
milk (1.0 mg)

Grains
raw flaxseed (4.9 mg)
raw granola (4.6 mg)
raw oatmeal (3.6 mg)
raw quinoa (3.0 mg)
wild rice (1.5 mg)
brown rice (0.7 mg)
white rice (0.6 mg)

Vegetables
mushrooms (0.6 mg)
spinach (0.6 mg)

Fruits
dried figs (0.6 micrograms)
dates (0.3 micrograms)

Beans
chickpeas (1.7 mg)
edamame (1.6 mg)
white beans (1.6 mg)
black-eyed peas (1.5 mg)
lentils (1.5 mg)
kidney beans (1.1 mg)
lima beans (1.1 mg)
navy beans (1.1 mg)
green beans (0.3 mg)

Other
chocolate (1.9 mg)
maple syrup (0.8 mg)

THE LETTERED VITAMINS

The lettered vitamins are essential nutrients for healthy body function.

Vitamin A

This nutrient helps regulate expression of genes and participates in a wide variety of activities within our cells. The recommended daily intake for vitamin A is between 4,000 and 10,000 IU per day. About 90 percent of this vitamin should come from beta-carotene instead of directly from vitamin A. Some of the best sources are (keeping in mind that these levels reflect beta-carotene conversion to vitamin A):

Vegetables	sweet potatoes (22,000 IU)	Beans	green beans (900 IU)
	carrots (19,000 IU)		
	kale (16,000 IU)	Fruit	cantaloupe (3,900 IU)
	spinach (11,000 IU)		apricots (2,200 IU)
	collard greens (9,300 IU)		grapefruit (1,400 IU)
	romaine lettuce (6,700 IU)		papaya (1,200 IU)
	basil (6,000 IU)		tomatoes (1,000 IU)
	squash (6,000 IU)		watermelon (700 IU)
	pumpkin (5,700 IU)		plums (400 IU)
	mint (4,800 IU)		blackberries (200 IU)
	sweet red peppers (3,700 IU)		
	red chile peppers (1,400 IU)	Dairy	cheddar cheese (1,100 IU)
	red cabbage (1,300 IU)		provolone (1,000 IU)
	green chile peppers (1,100 IU)		mozzarella (700 IU)
	scallions (1,100 IU)		eggs (600 IU)
	brussels sprouts (900 IU)		milk (200 IU)
	asparagus (900 IU)		
	broccoli (700 IU)	Fish	trout (300 IU)
	sweet green peppers (400 IU)		salmon (200 IU)
	okra (300 IU)		

Vitamin B1—Thiamine

This vitamin assists in the formation of energy, among other functions. The recommended daily dose of vitamin B1 is between 1.5 and 3.0 mg per day. Some of the best sources are:

Nuts	pistachios (1.0 mg)	cashews (0.5 mg)
	pine nuts (1.0 mg)	almonds (0.2 mg)
	pecans (0.8 mg)	chestnuts (0.2 mg)
	hazelnuts (0.7 mg)	walnuts (0.1 mg)
	peanuts (0.7 mg)	

Beans	navy beans (0.3 mg)	Fruits	dates (0.2 mg)
	black-eyed peas (0.2 mg)		dried figs (0.1 mg)
	edamame (0.2 mg)		oranges (0.1 mg)
	kidney beans (0.2 mg)		
	lentils (0.2 mg)	Meat/Fish	trout (0.3 mg)
	chickpeas (0.1 mg)		dark meat chicken (0.1 mg)
	green beans (0.1 mg)		chicken breast (0.1 mg)
	white beans (0.1 mg)		ground beef (0.05 mg)
			cod (0.03 mg)
Vegetables	artichoke (0.2 mg)		
	okra (0.2 mg)	Grains	raw flaxseed (1.9 mg)
	carrots (0.1 mg)		raw granola (0.8 mg)
			raw quinoa (0.4 mg)
			wheat bread (0.4 mg)
			raw oatmeal (0.3 mg)
			brown rice (0.1 mg)
		Dairy	milk (0.1 mg)

Vitamin B2—Riboflavin

This vitamin assists in the formation of energy, among other functions. The recommended daily dose of vitamin B2 is between 1.5 and 2.5 mg per day. One should be careful not to approach or exceed 10 mg per day. Some of the best sources are:

Meat/Fish	dark meat chicken (0.3 mg)		pistachios (0.2 mg)
	ground beef (0.2 mg)		walnuts (0.2 mg)
	salmon (0.2 mg)		
	chicken breast (0.1 mg)	Beans	edamame (0.2 mg)
	flounder (0.1 mg)		black-eyed peas (0.1 mg)
	cod (0.06 mg)		chickpeas (0.1 mg)
			green beans (0.1 mg)
Nuts	almonds (1.3 mg)		kidney beans (0.1 mg)
	cashews (0.3 mg)		lentils (0.1 mg)
	hazelnuts (0.2 mg)		lima beans (0.1 mg)
	peanuts (0.2 mg)		navy beans (0.1 mg)
	pecans (0.2 mg)		white beans (0.1 mg)
	pine nuts (0.2 mg)		

191

Grains	raw granola (0.3 mg)	**Fruits**	dried figs (0.7 mg)
	raw quinoa (0.3 mg)		dates (0.1 mg)
	raw flaxseed (0.2 mg)		
	raw oatmeal (0.1 mg)	**Dairy**	feta cheese (1.0 mg)
			eggs (0.6 mg)
Vegetables	mushrooms (0.5 mg)		yogurt (0.5 mg)
	mint (0.3 mg)		cheddar cheese (0.4 mg)
	spinach (0.2 mg)		mozzarella cheese (0.3 mg)
	squash (0.2 mg)		cottage cheese (0.2 mg)
	broccoli (0.1 mg)		milk (0.1 mg)
	brussels sprouts (0.1 mg)		

Vitamin B3—Niacin

Similar to some of the other B-complex vitamins, this nutrient also assists in the formation of energy, among other functions. The recommended daily dose of vitamin B3 is between 25 and 50 mg per day. Some of the best sources are:

Nuts	peanuts (15 mg)	**Beans**	lentils (1.2 mg)
	sunflower seeds (8.1 mg)		edamame (1.0 mg)
	almonds (4.0 mg)		green beans (0.7 mg)
	hazelnuts (2.0 mg)		kidney beans (0.7 mg)
	chestnuts (1.5 mg)		navy beans (0.7 mg)
	peanuts (1.5 mg)		chickpeas (0.6 mg)
	pistachios (1.5 mg)		black-eyed peas (0.5 mg)
	pecans (1.3 mg)		lima beans (0.5 mg)
	cashews (1.2 mg)		white beans (0.2 mg)
	walnuts (0.5 mg)		
		Vegetables	mushrooms (4.1 mg)
Meat/Fish	chicken breast (16.0 mg)		mint (1.9 mg)
	steak (9.5 mg)		asparagus (1.3 mg)
	dark meat chicken (8.0 mg)		red peppers (1.2 mg)
	salmon (7.7 mg)		artichoke (1.2 mg)
	ground beef (6.0 mg)		corn (1.2 mg)
	haddock (5.3 mg)		basil (1.0 mg)
	cod (2.9 mg)		
	crab (1.5 mg)	**Fruits**	dates (1.4 mg)
		Dairy	eggs (0.1 mg)
			cheese (0.1 mg)
			milk (0.1 mg)

Vitamin B6—Pyridoxine, Pyridoxal, and Pyridoxamine

This family of B-complex vitamins plays a central role in many enzymes and in energy production. The recommended daily dose of vitamin B6 is between 2 and 4 mg per day, and should not exceed 100 mg per day. Some of the best sources are:

Nuts
pine nuts (1.9 mg)
pistachios (1.9 mg)
walnuts (0.7 mg)
chestnuts (0.6 mg)
hazelnuts (0.6 mg)
cashews (0.5 mg)
peanuts (0.4 mg)
almonds (0.2 mg)
pecans (0.2 mg)

Meat/Fish
chicken breast (0.7 mg)
steak (0.6 mg)
turkey (0.5 mg)
cod (0.5 mg)
ground beef (0.4 mg)
salmon (0.3 mg)
crab (0.2 mg)

Vegetables
chile peppers (0.6 mg)
sweet potatoes (0.3 mg)
brussels sprouts (0.3 mg)
potatoes (0.3 mg)
spinach (0.3 mg)
cauliflower (0.2 mg)
broccoli (0.2 mg)
onions (0.2 gm)
corn (0.1 mg)
mint (0.1 mg)
mushrooms (0.1 mg)

Fruits
dates (0.2 mg)

Grains
raw flaxseed (0.5 mg)
raw quinoa (0.5 mg)
raw granola (0.3 mg)
raw oatmeal (0.3 mg)
brown rice (0.2 mg)

Dairy
cheddar cheese (0.1 mg)
cottage cheese (0.1 mg)
mozzarella cheese (0.1 mg)
milk (0.1 mg)

Vitamin B9—Folate or Folic Acid

This vitamin is essential for making DNA and proteins. The recommended daily dose of folate is between 800 and 1,000 micrograms per day. Levels up to about 5,000 micrograms per day are safe, but many doctors will urge patients not to take more than 1,000 micrograms per day for fear that the folate will mask a deficiency of vitamin B12. With a balanced diet that includes animal or dairy products (the sources for vitamin B12), the risk should be minimized. Some of the best sources are:

Nuts	peanuts (160 micrograms)		kidney beans (150 micrograms)
	hazelnuts (130 micrograms)		navy beans (150 micrograms)
	walnuts (120 micrograms)		lima beans (100 micrograms)
	chestnuts (80 micrograms)		white beans (100 micrograms)
	pine nuts (60 micrograms)		green beans (40 micrograms)
	pistachios (60 micrograms)		
	almonds (50 micrograms)	**Vegetables**	spinach (220 micrograms)
	cashews (50 micrograms)		asparagus (180 micrograms)
	pecans (50 micrograms)		lettuce (160 micrograms)
	walnuts (40 micrograms)		collard greens (110 micrograms)
			broccoli (70 micrograms)
Meats	ground beef (10 micrograms)		corn (70 micrograms)
			okra (50 micrograms)
Beans	edamame (350 micrograms)		
	black-eyed peas	**Grains**	white bread (180 micrograms)
	(200 micrograms)		white rice (120 micrograms)
	chickpeas (200 micrograms)		brown rice (5 micrograms)
	lentils (200 micrograms)		

Vitamin B12—Cobalamin

This essential vitamin removes the toxin homocystein, which we learned about in chapter 3 and is important in other cellular reactions. The recommended daily dose of vitamin B12 is between 5 and 20 micrograms per day. Vitamin B12 comes only from animal and dairy products (with rare exceptions). Some of the best sources are:

Meat/Fish	crab (14 micrograms)	**Dairy**	mozzarella cheese
	salmon (5.1 micrograms)		(2.5 micrograms)
	flounder (3.9 micrograms)		milk (1.2 micrograms)
	lobster (3.6 micrograms)		cottage cheese (0.8 micrograms)
	ground beef (3.2 micrograms)		yogurt (0.7 micrograms)
	shrimp (2.2 micrograms)		eggs (0.4 micrograms)
	cod (1.2 micrograms)		
		Other	white chocolate
			(0.8 micrograms)

Vitamin C—Ascorbate or Ascorbic Acid

This vitamin is involved in many enzyme reactions and assists in making collagen. The recommended daily dose of vitamin C is between 500 and 800 mg per day, and should not exceed 2,000 mg per day. Some of the best sources are:

Fruits		Vegetables	
Fruits	kiwis (100 mg)	Vegetables	red peppers (200 mg)
	strawberries (70 mg)		chile peppers (140 mg)
	papaya (70 mg)		green peppers (100 mg)
	oranges (60 mg)		broccoli (100 mg)
	grapefruit (40 mg)		brussels sprouts (70 mg)
	cantaloupe (40 mg)		cauliflower (50 mg)
	star fruit (40 mg)		spinach (32 mg)
	mangoes (30 mg)		okra (20 mg)
	raspberries (30 mg)		potatoes (13 mg)
	tomatoes (15 mg)		corn (8 mg)
	bananas (10 mg)		carrots (7 mg)
	watermelon (9 mg)		
	cherries (8 mg)	Beans	green beans (10 mg)
	peaches (8 mg)		
	apples (5 mg)	Nuts	chestnuts (45 mg)
	pears (5 mg)		hazelnuts (7 mg)
	grapes (5 mg)		pine nuts (6 mg)
	dried figs (1 mg)		pistachios (6 mg)
			walnuts (2 mg)
			pecans (1 mg)
		Fish	shrimp (2 mg)
			cod (1 mg)

Vitamin D—Calciferol or Calcitriol

This nutrient is actually not a vitamin but a steroid hormone that works to activate genes within the body. The recommended daily dose of vitamin D is between 200 and 800 IU per day, and should not exceed 2,000 IU per day. The human body can make its own vitamin D. Some of the best sources are:

Fish		Vegetables	
	herring (1,800 IU)		mushrooms (140 IU)
	salmon (700 IU)		
	catfish (580 IU)	Dairy	milk (100 IU)
	shrimp (180 IU)		eggs (60 IU)
	flounder (70 IU)		swiss cheese (50 IU)
	cod (50 IU)		parmesan cheese (32 IU)
			cheddar cheese (14 IU)

Vitamin E—Alpha-Tocopherol

This essential vitamin is a strong antioxidant and is important in other cellular reactions. The recommended daily dose of vitamin E is between 150 and 200 IU per day. Higher doses may cause bleeding complications. Some of the best sources are:

Nuts		Vegetables	
	sunflower seeds (44 IU)		spinach (3.5 IU)
	almonds (44 IU)		red peppers (2.8 IU)
	hazelnuts (26 IU)		asparagus (2.7 IU)
	pine nuts (16 IU)		pinto beans (1.6 IU)
	peanuts (13 IU)		kidney beans (1.5 IU)
	pistachios (3.9 IU)		broccoli (1.4 IU)
	pecans (2.4 IU)		carrots (1 IU)
	walnuts (1.2 IU)		green beans (0.8 IU)
			green peppers (0.7 IU)
Fish	herring (2.9 IU)		
	rockfish (2.7 IU)	Fruits	kiwis (2.5 IU)
	shrimp (1.9 IU)		blackberries (2 IU)
	lobster (1.7 IU)		mangoes (1.9 IU)
	cod (1.4 IU)		raspberries (1.6 IU)
	salmon (1.1 IU)		papaya (1.5 IU)
			peaches (1.3 IU)
Dairy	eggs (1.7 IU)		blueberries (1 IU)
			tomatoes (1 IU)

Vitamin K—Phylloquinone, Menaquinone, Menadione

This nutrient is essential for blood clotting and bone maintenance. The recommended daily dose of vitamin K is between 90 and 120 micrograms per day. Higher amounts of vitamin K may be recommended if one is taking higher amounts of vitamin E, omega-3 oils, or gingko—all of which increase susceptibility to bleeding. Some of the best sources are:

Vegetables
parsley (1,900 micrograms)
kale (950 micrograms)
spinach (570 micrograms)
beet greens (530 micrograms)
basil (470 micrograms)
scallions (240 micrograms)
broccoli (160 micrograms)
brussels sprouts
  (160 micrograms)
asparagus (60 micrograms)
okra (46 micrograms)
red cabbage (45 micrograms)
alfalfa (40 micrograms)
celery (35 micrograms)
cucumbers (19 micrograms)
pumpkin (18 micrograms)
cauliflower (18 micrograms)
artichoke (17 micrograms)
carrots (15 micrograms)

Beans
edamame (30 micrograms)
green beans (20 micrograms)

Fruits
blueberries (22 micrograms)
grapes (17 micrograms)

AMINO ACIDS

These nutrients are the building blocks of proteins.

Arginine

This amino acid regulates a gas called nitric oxide that affects blood vessel relaxation. The recommended minimum daily dose is 500 to 1,500 mg or more, but use caution if you are diabetic as excess amino acids are turned into sugars. Also, excess arginine can trigger reactivation of the herpes virus in someone who has a previous history of shingles or other herpes infection. Some of the best sources are:

Meat/Fish
- turkey breast (2,300 mg)
- steak (2,000 mg)
- ground beef (2,000 mg)
- shrimp (2,000 mg)
- flounder (1,700 mg)
- cod (1,600 mg)
- chicken breast (1,500 mg)

Nuts
- walnuts (4,000 mg)
- peanuts (3,500 mg)
- almonds (2,800 mg)
- hazelnuts (2,500 mg)
- cashews (2,400 mg)
- pine nuts (2,300 mg)
- pistachios (2,300 mg)
- pecans (1,300 mg)
- chestnuts (100 mg)

Dairy
- eggs (1,000 mg)
- cheese (1,000 mg)
- milk (100 mg)

Beans
- chickpeas (900 mg)
- edamame (800 mg)
- lentils (800 mg)
- white beans (700 mg)
- black-eyed peas (600 mg)
- kidney beans (500 mg)
- lima beans (500 mg)
- navy beans (500 mg)
- green beans (100 mg)

Vegetables
- broccoli (200 mg)
- spinach (200 mg)
- corn (200 mg)
- basil (130 mg)
- carrots (100 mg)
- okra (40 mg)

Fruit
- dates (150 mg)
- watermelon (70 mg)
- oranges (60 mg)
- mangoes (50 mg)
- cantaloupe (40 mg)
- peaches (40 mg)
- cherries (40 mg)
- strawberries (30 mg)
- tomatoes (30 mg)
- pears (20 mg)
- blueberries (20 mg)
- apples (10 mg)
- bananas (10 mg)

Grains
- raw flaxseed (2,200 mg)
- raw granola (1,500 mg)
- raw quinoa (1,100 mg)
- brown rice (700 mg)
- white bread (400 mg)
- white rice (300 mg)

Carnitine

This amino acid assists with many cellular enzymes. There is no minimum required dosing amount for carnitine; 20 to 500 mg per day may be sufficient, but use caution if you are diabetic as excess amino acids are turned into sugars. Some of the best sources are:

Meat/Fish	steak (110 mg)	**Dairy**	milk (7.5 mg)
	ground beef (110 mg)		American cheese (4.3 mg)
	cod (6.4 mg)		cottage cheese (3 mg)
	chicken breast (4.5 mg)		

Lysine

This amino acid is a building block of collagen. The recommended minimum daily dose is 800 to 1,200 mg, but use caution if you are diabetic as excess amino acids are turned into sugars. Some of the best sources are:

Meat/Fish	flounder (3,000 mg)	**Beans**	edamame (800 mg)
	steak (3,000 mg)		white beans (800 mg)
	turkey (3,000 mg)		chickpeas (700 mg)
	ground beef (2,500 mg)		kidney beans (700 mg)
	cod (2,400 mg)		lentils (700 mg)
	shrimp (2,000 mg)		black-eyed peas (600 mg)
	chicken breast (2,000 mg)		lima beans (600 mg)
			navy beans (600 mg)
Nuts	pistachios (1,300 mg)		
	pine nuts (1,300 mg)	**Vegetables**	spinach (200 mg)
	cashews (1,000 mg)		broccoli (200 mg)
	peanuts (1,000 mg)		corn (200 mg)
	walnuts (800 mg)		okra (100 mg)
	almonds (600 mg)		carrots (100 mg)
	hazelnuts (500 mg)		
	pecans (300 mg)	**Fruits**	oranges (60 mg)
	chestnuts (100 mg)		mangoes (50 mg)
			cherries (40 mg)
Dairy	cheese (2,200 mg)		cantaloupe (35 mg)
	eggs (1,000 mg)		peaches (35 mg)
	milk (120 mg)		tomatoes (30 mg)
		Grains	brown rice (350 mg)
			white bread (300 mg)
			wheat bread (200 mg)
			white rice (100 mg)

Methionine

This amino acid assists with many cellular enzymes including removal of debris from behind the retina. No ideal daily dose has been established. A concern is that excess methionine can result in buildup of the toxic chemical homocysteine. Perhaps a daily amount of 500 to 1,000 mg or somewhat more is acceptable, but use caution if you are diabetic as excess amino acids are turned into sugars. Some of the best sources are:

Meat/Fish	steak (900 mg)		edamame (100 mg)
	turkey (900 mg)		kidney beans (100 mg)
	flounder (800 mg)		lentils (100 mg)
	cod (800 mg)		lima beans (100 mg)
	shrimp (700 mg)		navy beans (100 mg)
	chicken breast (700 mg)		green beans (25 mg)
	ground beef (700 mg)		
		Vegetables	corn (80 mg)
Nuts	walnuts (500 mg)		spinach (60 mg)
	cashews (400 mg)		basil (40 mg)
	peanuts (400 mg)		broccoli (40 mg)
	pine nuts (400 mg)		mushrooms (40 mg)
	pistachios (400 mg)		carrots (20 mg)
	hazelnuts (250 mg)		okra (20 mg)
	almonds (200 mg)		
	pecans (200 mg)	**Grains**	raw flaxseed (400 mg)
	chestnuts (40 mg)		raw granola (300 mg)
			raw quinoa (300 mg)
Dairy	cheese (600 mg)		brown rice (200 mg)
	eggs (440 mg)		white bread (200 mg)
	milk (90 mg)		wheat bread (100 mg)
			white rice (80 mg)
Beans	white beans (150 mg)		
	black-eyed peas (100 mg)		
	chickpeas (100 mg)		

Proline

Although this nutrient is a building block of proteins, it is technically not an amino acid, though frequently classified with the amino acids. It plays a central role in making collagen. There is actually no established recommended dose and little is known about the ability of proline to be absorbed by the body after consuming foods with proline. Some of the best sources are:

Meat/Fish		Beans	
	steak (1,600 mg)		edamame (800 mg)
	ground beef (1,600 mg)		kidney beans (600 mg)
	turkey (1,500 mg)		navy beans (500 mg)
	chicken breast (1,300 mg)		white beans (500 mg)
	flounder (1,000 mg)		black-eyed peas (400 mg)
	cod (1,000 mg)		chickpeas (400 mg)
	shrimp (700 mg)		lentils (400 mg)
			lima beans (400 mg)
Nuts	peanuts (1,300 mg)		green beans (75 mg)
	almonds (1,100 mg)		
	walnuts (1,000 mg)	Vegetables	corn (300 mg)
	cashews (900 mg)		basil (120 mg)
	pine nuts (900 mg)		spinach (100 mg)
	pistachios (900 mg)		carrots (100 mg)
	hazelnuts (600 mg)		broccoli (100 mg)
	pecans (400 mg)		okra (100 mg)
	chestnuts (100 mg)		
		Grains	raw flaxseed (900 mg)
Dairy	cheese (2,300 mg)		raw granola (800 mg)
	eggs (600 mg)		raw quinoa (800 mg)
	milk (400 mg)		wheat bread (700 mg)
			brown rice (400 mg)
			white rice (200 mg)

Taurine

This amino acid is important for many activities; it decreases inflammation and transports vitamin A to the retina. There are no established clear dosing guidelines; a reasonable daily amount may be 50 to 500 mg, but use caution if you are diabetic as excess amino acids are turned into sugars. Some of the best sources are:

Meat/Fish		Dairy	milk (17 mg)
	flounder (198 mg)		
	steak (44 mg)		
	cod (34 mg)	Vegetables	seaweed (9 mg)
	chicken (17 mg)		
	ground beef (15 mg)		
	shrimp (13 mg)		

THE SPECIAL POWER NUTRIENTS

These nutrients play essential roles within cells.

Coenzyme Q10—Ubiquinone or Ubiquinol

This antioxidant nutrient plays a central role in helping mitochondria produce energy. The recommended daily dose is between 50 and 200 mg. It is best to divide the amount ingested per day into separate portions as very little of coenzyme Q10 is absorbed with each meal. Some of the best sources are:

Meat/Fish	sardines (74 mg)	**Vegetables**	spinach (12 mg)
	ground beef (36 mg)		broccoli (10 mg)
	chicken (24 mg)		green peppers (4 mg)
	flounder (6 mg)		sweet potatoes (4 mg)
			carrots (3 mg)
Nuts	peanuts (31 mg)		eggplant (2 mg)
	pistachios (24 mg)		cauliflower (2 mg)
	walnuts (23 mg)		cabbage (2 mg)
	hazelnuts (20 mg)		eggplant (2 mg)
	almonds (20 mg)		potatoes (1 mg)
			onions (1 mg)
Dairy	milk (18 mg)		
	eggs (4 mg)	**Beans**	green beans (68 mg)
	cheddar cheese (2 mg)		
		Grains	brown rice (6 mg)
			wheat germ (4 mg)
			buckwheat (2 mg)

Choline

This nutrient is tremendously important in forming cell-signaling molecules. There are no established clear dosing guidelines; a daily consumption of around 200 mg is often sufficient. Some of the best sources are:

Nuts	peanuts (120 mg)		**Meat/Fish**	ground beef (100 mg)
	cashews (70 mg)			cod (100 mg)
	almonds (60 mg)			shrimp (90 mg)
	pine nuts (60 mg)			steak (80 mg)
	hazelnuts (50 mg)			salmon (70 mg)
	pecans (45 mg)			chicken (6 mg)
	walnuts (40 mg)			
			Dairy	eggs (290 mg)
Vegetables	basil (13 mg)			milk (20 mg)
				cottage cheese (4 mg)
Fruits	dried figs (18 mg)			cheddar cheese (2 mg)
	dates (7 mg)			yogurt (2 mg)
Beans	edamame (60 mg)		**Grains**	raw flaxseed (90 mg)
	chickpeas (50 mg)			raw quinoa (70 mg)
	navy beans (50 mg)			raw granola (55 mg)
	black-eyed peas (40 mg)			bread (40 mg)
	lentils (40 mg)			raw oatmeal (30 mg)
	lima beans (40 mg)			brown rice (10 mg)
	white beans (40 mg)			
	kidney beans (30 mg)			
	green beans (20 mg)			

SAMe

This nutrient helps prevent DNA damage and performs other important functions inside our cells. SAMe is not found in foods because it is unstable at room temperatures. The human body makes its own SAMe. A healthy balanced diet filled with folate-rich foods may be the best approach to increasing SAMe levels in your body.

FISH OILS

DHA is one of the most important of the omega-3 oils.

DHA

This omega-3 oil forms membranes of the retinal cells, particularly the light-sensing photoreceptors, and performs many other functions such as turning on genes involved in growth and survival of cells as well as blocking inflammation. An averaged daily dose (averaged over the course of a week) of around 500 mg per day is reasonable, along with other omega-3 oils. For most people, the total daily dose of omega-3 oils should not exceed 3,000 mg per day. Some of the best sources are:

Meat/Fish	salmon (1,600 mg)	Dairy	eggs (50 mg)
	sardines (1,500 mg)		American cheese (10 mg)
	trout (600 mg)		
	anchovy (600 mg)	Grains	raw quinoa (50 mg)
	rockfish (150 mg)		
	shrimp (150 mg)		
	chicken (80 mg)		
	turkey (50 mg)		

SELECTED BIBLIOGRAPHY

Age-Related Eye Disease Study 2 Research Group. "Lutein + Zeaxanthin and Omega-3 Fatty Acids for Age-Related Macular Degeneration: the Age-Related Eye Disease Study 2 (AREDS2) Randomized Clinical Trial." *JAMA* 309 (2013): 2005–15.

Age-Related Eye Disease Study Research Group. "A Randomized, Placebo-Controlled Clinical Trial of High-Dose Supplementation with Vitamins C and E, Beta Carotene, and Zinc for Age-Related Macular Degeneration and Vision Loss: AREDS Report No. 8." *Arch Ophthalmol* 119 (2001): 1417–36.

———. "A Randomized, Placebo-Controlled, Clinical Trial of High-Dose Supplementation with Vitamins C and E and Beta Carotene for Age-Related Cataract and Vision Loss: AREDS Report No. 9." *Arch Ophthalmol* 119 (2001): 1439–52.

Age-Related Macular Degeneration Study Group. "Multicenter Ophthalmic and Nutritional Age-Related Macular Degeneration Study—Part 2: Antioxidant Intervention and Conclusions." *J Am Optom Assoc* 67 (1996): 30–49.

Amirul Islam, F. M., E. W. Chong, A. M. Hodge, et al. "Dietary Patterns and Their Associations with Age-Related Macular Degeneration: The Melbourne Collaborative Cohort Study." *Ophthalmology* 121 (2014): 1428–34.

Aslam, T., C. Delcourt, R. Silva, et al. "Micronutrients in Age-Related Macular Degeneration." *Ophthalmologica* 229 (2013): 75–9.

Beatty, S., U. Chakravarthy, J. M. Nolan, et al. "Secondary Outcomes in a Clinical Trial of Carotenoids with Coantioxidants versus Placebo in Early Age-Related Macular Degeneration." *Ophthalmology* 120 (2013): 600–6.

Berson, E. L., B. Rosner, M. A. Sandberg, et al. "A Randomized Trial of Vitamin A and Vitamin E Supplementation for Retinitis Pigmentosa." *Arch Ophthalmol* 111 (1993): 761–72.

———. "Clinical Trial of Lutein in Patients with Retinitis Pigmentosa Receiving Vitamin A." *Arch Ophthalmol* 128 (2010): 403–11.

———. "Ω-3 Intake and Visual Acuity in Patients with Retinitis Pigmentosa Receiving Vitamin A." *Arch Ophthalmol* 130 (2012): 707–11.

———. "Clinical Trial of Docosahexaenoic Acid in Patients with Retinitis Pigmentosa Receiving Vitamin A Treatment." *Arch Ophthalmol* 122 (2004): 1297–1305.

———. "Further Evaluation of Docosahexaenoic Acid in Patients with Retinitis Pigmentosa Receiving Vitamin A Treatment." *Arch Ophthalmol* 122 (2004): 1306–14.

Brignole-Baudouin, F., C. Baudouin, P. Aragona, et al. "A Multicentre, Double-Masked, Randomized, Controlled Trial Assessing the Effect of Oral Supplementation of Omega-3 and Omega-6 Fatty Acids on a Conjunctival Inflammatory Marker in Dry Eye Patients." *Acta Ophthalmol* 89 (2011): e591–7.

Brown, L., E. B. Rimm, J. M. Seddon, et al. "A Prospective Study of Carotenoid Intake and Risk of Cataract Extraction in US Men." *Am J Clin Nutr* 70 (1999): 517–24.

Chasan-Taber, L., W. C. Willett, J. M. Seddon, et al. "A Prospective Study of Vitamin Supplement Intake and Cataract Extraction among US Women." *Epidemiology* 10 (1999): 679.

Chew, E. "Vitamins and Minerals, for Eyes Only?" *JAMA Ophthalmol* 132 (2014): 665–6.

Cho, E., J. M. Seddon, B. Rosner, et al. "Prospective Study of Intake of Fruits, Vegetables, Vitamins, and Carotenoids and Risk of Age-Related Maculopathy." *Arch Ophthalmol* 122 (2004): 883–92.

Cho, E., M. J. Stampfer, J. M. Seddon, et al. "Prospective Study of Zinc Intake and the Risk of Age-Related Macular Degeneration." *Ann Epidemiol* 11 (2001): 328–36.

Christen, W. G., R. J. Glynn, E. Y. Chew, et al. "Folic Acid, Pyridoxine, and Cyanocobalamin Combination Treatment and Age-Related Macular Degeneration in Women: the Women's Antioxidant and Folic Acid Cardiovascular Study." *Arch Intern Med* 169 (2009): 335–41.

Christen, W. G., R. J. Glynn, H. D. Sesso, et al. "Vitamins E and C and Medical Record–Confirmed Age-Related Macular Degeneration in a Randomized Trial of Male Physicians." *Ophthalmology* 119 (2012): 1642–9.

Christen, W. G., R. J. Glynn, J. E. Manson, et al. "Effects of Multivitamin Supplement on Cataract and Age-Related Macular Degeneration in a Randomized Trial of Male Physicians." *Ophthalmology* 121 (2014): 525–34.

Christen, W. G., R. J. Glynn, R. D. Sperduto, et al. "Age-Related Cataract in a Randomized Trial of Beta-Carotene in Women." *Ophthalmic Epidemiol* 11 (2004): 401–12.

Christen, W. G., J. E. Manson, R. J. Glynn, et al. "A Randomized Trial of Beta Carotene and Age-Related Cataract in US Physicians." *Arch Ophthalmol* 121 (2003): 372–8.

Chylack, L.T., Jr., N. P. Brown, A. Bron, et al. "The Roche European American Cataract Trial (REACT): a Randomized Clinical Trial to Investigate the Efficacy of an Oral Antioxidant Micronutrient Mixture to Slow Progression of Age-Related Cataract." *Ophthalmic Epidemiol* 9 (2002): 49–80.

Cumming, R. G., P. Mitchell, and W. Smith. "Diet and Cataract: the Blue Mountains Eye Study." *Ophthalmology* 107 (2000): 450–6.

Dagnelie, G., I. S. Zorge, and T. M. McDonald. "Lutein Improves Visual Function in Some Patients with Retinal Degeneration: a Pilot Study via the Internet." *Optometry* 71 (2000): 147–64.

Dasch, B., A. Fuhs, J. Schmidt, et al. "Serum Levels of Macular Carotenoids in Relation to Age-Related Maculopathy. The Muenster Aging and Retina Study (MARS)." *Graefes Arch Clin Exp Ophthalmol* 243 (2005): 1028–35.

Delcourt, C., J. P. Cristol, F. Tessier, et al. "Age-Related Macular Degeneration and Antioxidant Status in the POLA Study. POLA Study Group. Pathologies Oculaires Liees a l'Age." *Arch Ophthalmol* 117 (1999): 1384–90.

Evans, J. R., and J. G. Lawrenson. "Antioxidant Vitamin and Mineral Supplements for Preventing Age-Related Macular Degeneration." *Cochrane Database Syst Rev* 13 (2012): 6.

———. "Antioxidant Vitamin and Mineral Supplements for Slowing the Progression of Age-Related Macular Degeneration." *Cochrane Database Syst Rev* 14 (2012): 11.

Feher, J., B. Kovacs, I. Kovacs, et al. "Improvement of Visual Functions and Fundus Alterations in Early Age-Related Macular Degeneration Treated with a Combination of Acetyl-L-Carnitine, n-3 Fatty Acids, and Coenzyme Q10." *Ophthalmologica* 219 (2005): 154–66.

Feher, J., A. Papale, G. Mannino, et al. "Mitotropic Compounds for the Treatment of Age-Related Macular Degeneration. The Metabolic Approach and a Pilot Study." *Ophthalmologica* 217 (2003): 351–7.

Flood, V., W. Smith, J. J. Wang, et al. "Dietary Antioxidant Intake and Incidence of Early Age-Related Maculopathy: the Blue Mountain Eye Study." *Ophthalmology* 109 (2002): 2272–8.

Glacet-Bernard, A., G. Coscas, A. Chabanel, et al. "A Randomized, Double-Masked Study on the Treatment of Retinal Vein Occlusion with Troxerutin." *Am J Ophthalmol* 118 (1994): 421–9.

Gopinath, B., V. M. Flood, E. Rochtchina, et al. "Homocysteine, Folate, Vitamin B-12, and 10-y Incidence of Age-Related Macular Degeneration." *Am J Clin Nutr* 98 (2013): 129–35.

Guallar, E., S. Stranges, C. Mulrow, et al. "Enough Is Enough: Stop Wasting Money on Vitamins and Mineral Supplements." *Ann Intern Med* 159 (2013): 850–1.

Hankinson, S. E., M. J. Stampfer, J. M. Seddon, et al. "Nutrient Intake and Cataract Extraction in Women: a Prospective Study." *BMJ* 305 (1992): 335–39.

Heuberger, R.A., J. A. Mares-Perlman, R. Klein, et al. "Relationship of Dietary Fat to Age-Related Maculopathy in the Third National Health and Nutrition Examination Survey." *Arch Ophthalmol* 119 (2001): 1833–8.

Hoffman, D. R., K. G. Locke, D. H. Wheaton, et al. "A Randomized, Placebo-Controlled Clinical Trial of Docosahexaenoic Acid Supplementation for x-linked Retinitis Pigmentosa." *Am J Ophthalmol* 137 (2004): 704–18.

Jacques, P. F., L. T. Chylack Jr., S. E. Hankinson, et al. "Long-Term Nutrient Intake and Early Age-Related Nuclear Lens Opacities." *Arch Ophthalmol* 119 (2001): 1009–19.

Jacques P. F., A. Taylor, S. E. Hankinson, et al. "Long-Term Vitamin C Supplement Use and Prevalence of Early Age-Related Lens Opacities." *Am J Clin Nutr* 66 (1997): 911–6. Companion study: Taylor, A., P. F. Jacques, L. T. Chylack Jr., et al. "Long-Term Intake of Vitamins and Carotenoids and Odds of Early Age-Related Cortical and Posterior Subcapsular Lens Opacities." *Am J Clin Nutr* 75 (2002): 540–49.

Krishnadev, N., A. D. Meleth, and E. Y. Chew. Nutritional Supplements for Age-Related Macular Degeneration. *Curr Opin Ophthalmol* 21 (2010): 184–9.

Kuzniarz, M., P. Mitchell, R. G. Cumming, and V. M. Flood. "Use of Vitamin Supplements and Cataract: the Blue Mountains Eye Study." *Am J Ophthalmol* 132 (2001): 19–26.

Kuzniarz, M., P. Mitchell, V. M. Flood, and J. J. Wang. "Use of Vitamin and Zinc Supplements and Age-Related Maculopathy: the Blue Mountains Eye Study." *Ophthalmic Epidemiol* 9 (2002): 283–95.

Leske, M. C., L. T. Chylack Jr., Q. He, et al. "Antioxidant Vitamins and Nuclear Opacities: the Longitudinal Study of Cataract." *Ophthalmology* 105 (1998): 831–6.

Lillico, A., B. Jacobs, M. Reid, et al. "Selenium Supplementation and Risk of Glaucoma in the NPC Trial Selenium and Cancer Projects Group." Tucson, AZ: Arizona Cancer Center, University of Arizona, 2002.

Lyle, B. J., J. A. Mares-Perlman, B. E. Klein, et al. "Antioxidant Intake and Risk of Incident Age-Related Nuclear Cataracts in the Beaver Dam Eye Study." *Am J Epidemiol* 149 (1999): 801.

Ma, L., H. L. Dou, Y. M. Huang, et al. "Improvement of Retinal Function in Early Age-Related Macular Degeneration after Lutein and Zeaxanthin Supplementation: a Randomized, Double-Masked, Placebo Controlled Trial." *Am J Ophthalmol* 154 (2012): 625–34.

Mares-Perlman, J. A., B. J. Lyle, R. Klein, et al. "Vitamin Supplement Use and Incident Cataracts in a Population-Based Study." *Arch Ophthalmol* 118 (2000): 1556–63.

Mares-Perlman, J. A., R. Klein, B. E. Klein, et al. "Association of Zinc and Antioxidant Nutrients with Age-Related Maculopathy." *Arch Ophthalmol* 114 (1996): 991–7.

Mares-Perlman, J. A., W. E. Brady, B. E. Klein, et al. "Diet and Nuclear Lens Opacities." *Am J Epidemiol* 141 (1995): 322–34.

Miljanovic, B., K. A. Trivedi, M. R. Dana, et al. "Relation between Dietary n-3 and n-6 Fatty Acids and Clinically Diagnosed Dry Eye Syndrome in Women." *Am J Clin Nutr* 82 (2005): 887–93.

Morales-Pasantes, H., H. Quiroz, and O. Quesada. "Treatment with Taurine, Diltiazem, and Vitamin E Retards the Progressive Visual Field Reduction in Retinitis Pigmentosa: a 3-Year Follow-Up Study." *Metab Brain Dis* 17 (2002): 183–97.

Pagliarini, S., A. Moramarco, R. P. Wormald, et al. "Age-Related Macular Disease in Rural Southern Italy." *Arch Ophthalmol* 115 (1997): 616–22.

Rautiainen, S., B. E. Lindblad, R. Morgenstern, et al. "Vitamin C Supplements and the Risk of Age-Related Cataract: a Population-Based Prospective Cohort Study in Women." *Am J Clin Nutr* 91 (2010): 487–93.

Reccia, R., B. Pignalosa, A. Grasso, and G. Campanella. "Taurine Treatment in Retinitis Pigmentosa." *Acta Neurol* 2 (1980): 132–36.

Rejdak, R., J. Toczolowski, J. Kurkowski, et al. "Oral Citicoline Treatment Improves Visual Pathway Function in Glaucoma." *Med Sci Monit* 9 (2003): PI24–28.

Richer, S., W. Stiles, L. Statkute, et al. "Double-Masked, Placebo-Controlled, Randomized Trial of Lutein and Antioxidant Supplementation in the Intervention of Atrophic Age-Related Macular Degeneration: the Veterans LAST study (Lutein Antioxidant Supplementation Trial)." *Optometry* 75 (2004): 216–30.

Seddon, J. M., U. A. Ajani, R. D. Sperduto, et al. "Dietary Carotenoids, Vitamins A, C, and E, and Advanced Age-Related Macular Degeneration." *JAMA* 272 (1994): 1413–20.

Seddon, J. M., W. G. Christen, J. E. Manson, et al. "The Use of Vitamin Supplements and the Risk of Cataract among US Male Physicians." *Am J Public Health* 84 (1994): 788–92.

Seddon, J. M., S. George, and B. Rosner. "Cigarette Smoking, Fish Consumption, Omega-3 Fatty Acid Intake, and Associations with Age-Related Macular Degeneration. The US Twin Study of Age-Related Macular Degeneration." *Arch Ophthalmol* 124 (2006): 995–1001.

Sperduto, R. D., T. S. Hu, R. C. Milton, et al. "The Linxian Cataract Studies. Two Nutrition Intervention Trials." *Arch Ophthalmol* 111 (1993): 1246–53.

Stough, C., L. Downey, B. Silber, et al. "The Effects of 90-Day Supplementation with the Omega-3 Essential Fatty Acid Docosahexaenoic Acid (DHA) on Cognitive Function and Visual Acuity in a Healthy Aging Population." *Neurobiol Aging* 33 (2012): 824.e1-3.

Tavani, A., E. Negri, and C. La Vecchia. "Food and Nutrient Intake and Risk of Cataract." *Ann Epidemiol* 6 (1996): 41–6.

Teikari, J. M., L. Laatikainen, J. Virtamo, et al. "Six-Year Supplementation with Alpha-Tocopherol and Beta-Carotene and Age-Related Maculopathy." *Acta Ophthalmol Scand* 76 (1998): 224–29.

Teikari, J. M., J. Virtamo, M. Rautalahti, et al. "Long-Term Supplementation with Alpha-Tocopherol and Beta-Carotene and Age-Related Cataract." *Acta Ophthalmol Scand* 75 (1997): 634–40.

Van Leeuwen, R., S. Boekhoorn, J. R. Vingerling, et al. "Dietary Intake of Antioxidants and Risk of Age-Related Macular Degeneration." *JAMA* 294 (2005): 3101–7.

VandenLangenberg, G. M., J. A. Mares-Perlman, R. Klein, et al. "Associations between Antioxidant and Zinc Intake and the 5 Year Incidence of Early Age-Related Maculopathy in the Beaver Dam Eye Study." *Am J Epidemiol* 148 (1998): 204–14.

Virno, M., J. Pecori-Giraldi, A. Liguori, and F. De Gregorio. "The Protective Effect of Citicoline on the Progression of the Perimetric Defects in Glaucomatous Patients (Perimetric Study with a 10-Year Follow-Up)." *Acta Ophthalmol Scand Suppl* 232 (2000): 56–7.

West, S., S. Vitale, J. Hallfrisch, et al. "Are Antioxidants or Supplements Protective for Age-Related Macular Degeneration?" *Arch Ophthalmol* 112 (1994): 222–7.

Wilkinson, J. T., and F. W. Fraunfelder. "Use of Herbal Medicines and Nutritional Supplements in Ocular Disorders: an Evidence-Based Review." *Drugs* 71 (2011): 2421–34.

Zwart, S. R., C. R. Gibson, T. H. Mader, et al. "Vision Changes after Spaceflight Are Related to Alterations in Folate- and Vitamin B-12-Dependent One-Carbon Metabolism." *J Nutr* 142 (2012): 427–31.

INDEX

ABOUT THE AUTHOR

Neal A. Adams, MD is a leading expert in ophthalmology. He is editor-in-chief of a peer-reviewed medical journal in his field, *Eye Reports,* and has served as chief of the Division of Visual Physiology at the Wilmer Eye Institute of the Johns Hopkins Hospital and chair of the Department of Ophthalmology at the Paul L. Foster School of Medicine at Texas Tech University. Dr. Adams has received many honors as a highly skilled surgeon and clinician. He has coined a new category of eye conditions called the "retinal ciliopathies." His private clinical practice in suburban Washington, DC, focuses on providing patients with medical, surgical, and nutrition-based care. Visit him at www.dcretina.com.